The Mediterranean Diet Cookbook

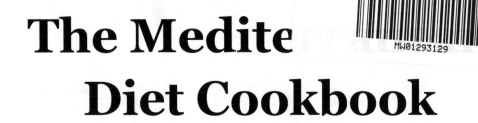

Delicious and Healthy Recipes for Natural Weight Loss with 7-Day Mediterranean Diet Meal Plan

Written by: Jolene Daisy

Copyright © 2018

All rights reserved.

All rights Reserved. No part of this publication or the information in it may be quoted from or reproduced in any form by means such as printing, scanning, photocopying or otherwise without prior written permission of the copyright holder.

Disclaimer and Terms of Use:

Effort has been made to ensure that the information in this book is accurate and complete, however, the author and the publisher do not warrant the accuracy of the information, text and graphics contained within the book due to the rapidly changing nature of science, research, known and unknown facts and internet. The Author and the publisher do not hold any responsibility for errors, omissions or contrary interpretation of the subject matter herein. This book is presented solely for motivational and informational purposes only. Please always consult a licensed professional before making changes to your lifestyle or diet.

Dedication

I dedicate this book to my family.

Table of Contents

INTRODUCTION 5
   Philosophy of the Mediterranean Diet 5
   The Origin of the Mediterranean Diet 6
   Food Pyramid of the Mediterranean Diet 6
   Health Benefits of the Mediterranean Diet 9
   Tips: How to Start the Mediterranean Diet 11

CHAPTER 1: MEDITERRANEAN APPETIZERS RECIPES 13
   Sandwiches with Cheese, Salad, Olives, and Grapes 13
   Stuffed Tomatoes 14
   Eggplant Rolls Stuffed with Cream Cheese and Tomatoes 15
   Mushrooms Stuffed with Cheese, Pepper, and Garlic 16
   Greek Yogurt Dip 17

CHAPTER 2: MEDITERRANEAN SALADS RECIPES 18
   Caprese Salad 18
   Salad with Fresh Spinach, Tuna, and Feta Cheese 19
   Fresh Green Salad with Shrimps and Avocado 20
   Salad with Fish and Fresh Vegetables 21
   Red Beans and Greens Salad 22
   Bulgur salad 23
   Colorful Vegetable Salad 24

CHAPTER 3: MEDITERRANEAN VEGETABLE RECIPES 25
   Sautéed Greek Zucchini 25
   Stuffed Eggplant with Fried Vegetables 26
   Vegetarian Mushroom Casserole 27
   Moroccan Style Vegetable Stew 28
   Mediterranean Chickpea Patties 29
   Braised Leeks 30

CHAPTER 4: MEDITERRANEAN SEAFOOD RECIPES 31
   Salmon Skewers with Pepper and Spices 31
   Baked Salmon with Vegetables Ratatouille 32
   Salmon Steak Fillet with Cheese Crust Breading 33
   Crispy Grilled Salmon Steak 34
   Grilled Tuna Steak with Red wine Sauce 35
   Grilled Sea Bass with Parsley and Lemon 36

    Shrimps and Vegetables Stir-Fry 37
    Shrimps with Asparagus, Tomatoes, and Paprika 38
    Baked Salmon with Lemon and Cherry Tomatoes 39
    Roasted Garlic Butter Salmon 40

CHAPTER 5: MEDITERRANEAN GRAINS AND LEGUMES RECIPES 41

    Garbanzos Greek Hummus 41
    Oatmeal with Strawberry 42
    Baked Beans 43
    Seafood Paella 44
    Quinoa Heaven 45
    Couscous Delight 46

CHAPTER 6: MEDITERRANEAN PASTA (MACARONI) RECIPES 47

    Penne Pasta with Pumpkin and Chili 47
    Mediterranean Macaroni and Cheese 48
    Chicken and Macaroni Baked 49
    Vermicelli Pudding 50
    Baked Macaroni with Broccoli 51
    Mediterranean Carbonara 52
    Pasta Salad 53

CHAPTER 7: MEDITERRANEAN MEAT AND POULTRY RECIPES 54

    Grilled Turkey Fillets 54
    Stuffed Peppers with Meat, Rice, and Vegetables 55
    Delicious Chicken Breasts with Lemon 56
    Roasted Lamb with Vegetables 57
    Pan Fried Pork Chops with Orange Sauce 58
    Mediterranean Meatballs in Tomato Sauce 59

CHAPTER 8: MEDITERRANEAN DESSERTS RECIPES 60

    Honey Glazed Apple 60
    Honey-Nuts Baked Pears 61
    Strawberry Chocolate Dip 62
    Vegan Blueberry Vanilla Smoothie 63

CHAPTER 9: 7-DAY MEDITERRANEAN DIET MEAL PLAN TO LOSE WEIGHT 64

CONCLUSION 72

Introduction

Philosophy of the Mediterranean Diet

Living healthy is an essential part of everyday life. Living in a world where everyone needs to be fit to survive is indeed a goal that everyone wants to achieve. Looking around in today's world, obesity, diabetes, cancer and heart diseases are at their all-time high.

Research has shown that Mediterranean foods, in fact, reduce the risk of these diseases. The Mediterranean style of eating focuses on natural foods such as fruits, veggies, nuts, and whole grains; fish and poultry; very limited red meat; using olive oil instead of butter; cooking with natural herbs and spices instead of salt and drinking red wine once in a while.

The Mediterranean diet isn't actually a "diet." Yes, it can help you lose weight and improve your health, but it's really more of a lifestyle. It's a way of eating that can keep you healthy and provide all the nutrients you need to live life to the fullest.

For the Mediterranean people, food encompasses cultural as well as ethical and historical values. In other words, food is considered a pleasure.

This "pleasure" is all about sharing food, socializing and spending time with others. In the Mediterranean culture, sharing meals together has always meant serenity and contentment. Food is seen as both a delight and an important societal act.

The Mediterranean culture is connected via the marketplace, the street, the church, the pub and the square where people meet and share their lives and thoughts with each other.

Eating together is a cheerful act that strengthens relationships, promotes relaxation and release, lessens stress and creates social harmony. The act of cooking a meal, then setting the table and serving food is a way of life that gives importance to people and pleases the senses with flavors, smells, colors, rhythms, and images that are imbued with the Mediterranean spirit.

Mediterranean people just know how to slow down and enjoy life and enjoy the food. North Americans don't value this as they should. Fast-food restaurants, fast-paced lives, and materialism have overrun this simple principle of healthy living.

The Origin of the Mediterranean Diet

This diet is based on the traditional dietary patterns of the countries that border the Mediterranean Sea such as Spain, Greece, Israel, Southern Italy and France. It gained widespread popularity in the west during the 1990's and since then has become one of the well-respected diets, particularly for its heart health and longevity benefits.

There are 21 countries that border the Mediterranean Sea; and though their diets, culture, agriculture, ethnic background and economy vary, there are common dietary patterns that they share. These common patterns have become characteristic of what we call the Mediterranean diet.

The most authentic version of the Mediterranean diet is based on the typical dietary patterns of the people of Crete (the largest Greek island) during the 1950's and 60's.

Food Pyramid of the Mediterranean Diet

The Mediterranean diet pyramid provides a general sense of the proportions and frequency of food group servings that make up the dietary pattern of Mediterranean.

The Mediterranean diet food pyramid helps you make wise choices. Plus, it's simple to follow. At the bottom of the pyramid are common staple foods that are to be consumed in large amounts and more frequently. Portion sizes and frequency decline as you go up the pyramid.

The pyramid is not a strict guide to recommended weights of foods or calories. It is just an overall look at wide variety of choices and idea of relative proportions that you can take as you come along with the specified allowances per category.

Moderation is the key

The Mediterranean diet encourages moderation and wise choices when it comes to food. For example, it's fine to enjoy a small piece of cake on occasion or a slice of steak with a glass of wine with friends and family because that's part of being human. The key is to be wise about the frequency and quantity of what you eat.

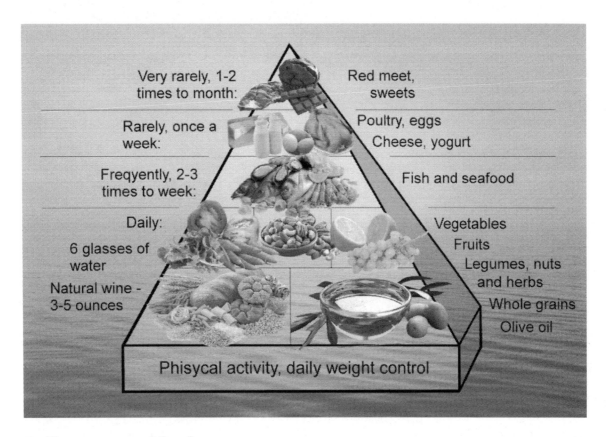

Daily consumed foods

Here are some of the daily foods that you can consume as suggested in the pyramid: whole grains, olive oil, vegetables, legumes, seeds, beans, nuts, herbs and spices (instead of salt), and fruits.

Frequently consumed foods

There are foods that you can take at least 2-3 times a week and mostly: fish and seafood – they are rich in iodine, which helps with proper thyroid metabolism and maintenance of weight.

Fish is the most common type of meat eaten on the Mediterranean diet and is typically consumed two to three times a week up to five or six times (including a variety of seafood as well as fish).

Rarely consumed foods

There is food that recommended to be consumed at least once a week like cheese, yogurt, poultry, and eggs due to their high-fat content. Animal fat is known to clog arteries and damage our cardiovascular health.

The biggest and most important difference to keep in mind is that Mediterranean dairy products are not made from cow's milk; rather they are made from sheep, buffalo or goats milk. Sheep and goat's milk have a lower amount of animal fat in them.

Very rarely consumed foods

Red meat and sweets should be consumed very rarely due to their adverse effect on health. Too much sweet is known to cause tooth decay and diabetes while red meat is much harder to digest and process by the body.

Stay hydrated

On the Mediterranean diet, you should drink 6-8 glasses of water, or about 60-70 ounces of water a day. It is highly recommended on the Mediterranean diet in order to stay hydrated as you flush toxins out of your body.

Drinking plenty of water also flushes your kidneys and bowels and keeps your skin looking younger.

Wine in moderation

Some research studies suggest that consuming red wine in moderation can reduce the risk of heart disease.

In the Mediterranean diet pyramid, a moderate amount of wine, typically one or two 5-ounce glasses of red wine served daily with a meal is suggested for men.

One glass of red wine served with a meal is suggested for women.

Exercise

Daily exercise is a very important part of the Mediterranean diet. Regular daily exercise (30 minutes a day) strengthens the cardiovascular system, builds muscle, boosts the immune system, maintains healthy bone density and joint mobility and releases myokines that promote tissue repair, the growth of new tissue and anti-inflammatory functions that help prevent diseases caused by inflammation.

Exercise also helps to prevent Type 2 diabetes, heart disease, cardiovascular disease, and obesity. It also enables your body to burn calories which reduces body mass index levels.

HEALTH BENEFITS OF THE MEDITERRANEAN DIET

The Mediterranean diet in its most holistic and authentic form includes more than just food. It is an approach to eating and to life that involves taking the time to enjoy both.

Here are some of the health benefits of the Mediterranean diet:

Preventing cardiovascular disease and strokes

Following the Mediterranean diet, you should limit to take refined bread and red meat. It encourages you to drink red wine which is helpful for proper blood circulation.

Reducing the risk of Alzheimer's

According to studies, Mediterranean diet helps to improve blood sugar and overall cholesterol level and helps the brain to enhance its memory.

Cutting the risk of Parkinson's disease

The Mediterranean diet helps in sustaining cells and prevents them from undergoing damage process, thus cutting the tendency of developing Parkinson's disease by 70%.

Protecting against type 2 diabetes

A Mediterranean diet is rich in fiber which helps in proper digestion and maintenance of sugar level.

Reducing the risk of cancer

Nowadays the food we eat affects us in so many ways. Foods rich in fiber and less salt is an ideal way to prevent cancer.

Increasing energy levels

Mediterranean diet is rich in fiber and essential nutrients that are necessary for daily body functioning. The more you consume high-fiber foods, the more your body will be forced to consume the stored fats in your body, thus increasing the reserved energy levels.

Regulating metabolic processes

There are studies suggesting that people who adhere to Mediterranean diet have better regulation of certain enzymes that affect the storage of fats. These enzymes are necessary for breaking down unnecessary fats in your body. Due to the fact that this diet is rich in antioxidant properties, it gives the body a better "engine" to perform.

Keeping you agile

It also reduces muscle weakness because the nutrients help you to sustain day-to-day activities.

Increasing longevity

Mediterranean people have mastered the art of enjoying and appreciating the gifts of nature, delighting in foods, enjoying the company of others and enjoying life itself. This quality enhances their health and increases their longevity.

Thus, the Mediterranean diet is an ideal for health-conscious individuals who would like to keep their body fit and healthy.

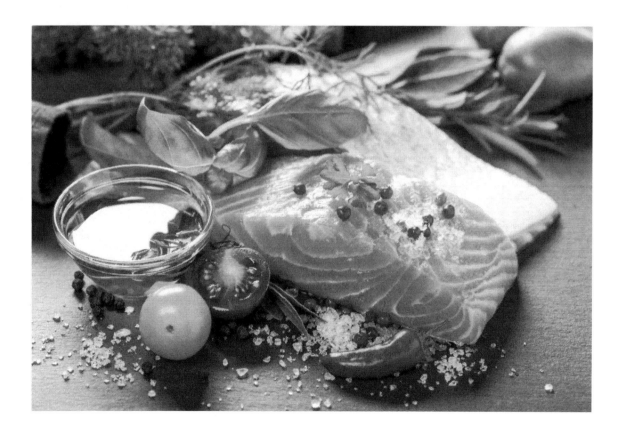

TIPS: HOW TO START THE MEDITERRANEAN DIET

If you are interested in applying the Mediterranean diet to your life to lose weight, then these general dieting tips paired with the Mediterranean diet eating habits will help you maximize your weight loss.

Use good unsaturated fats

Good fats come mainly from vegetables, nuts, seeds, and fish.

Replace butter and margarine with olive oil. I especially like to use olive oil when grilling sandwiches or toasting bread where at one time I only used butter or margarine.

Keep a jar of mixed nuts on your kitchen counter and eat a handful of those along with your *vegetable* or fruit snack.

Eat more vegetable-based meals

The Mediterranean Diet encourages eating an abundance of fresh vegetables and fruits. This is another great opportunity to try some new spices mixed with cooked vegetables, legumes or in a vegetable dip.

Change your thinking on vegetables and turn them into snacks in the middle of the day or get in the habit of having a vegetable platter on the table during dinner. Drizzle some olive oil over the vegetables before diving in. And put a small bowl of nuts and seeds besides the vegetable platter so you can munch on those along with the vegetables.

Have a salad with every meal. Be creative and top your greens with all kinds of colorful vegetables, nuts, seeds, herbs and even a sliced egg. Make a simple olive oil and lemon dressing and drizzle it over your salad.

Many Mediterranean households typically have a vegetable garden and fruit trees in their yard. Even people that live in cities have window boxes in which they grow their own foods.

Eat vegetables and fruits as snacks

Slice your vegetables into ready-to-eat snack sizes and wash your fruits when you bring them home from the store so that they are ready to grab as a quick snack when you're feeling hungry.

Split your plate into three sections

Visually split your plate in half then split one of those halves in two. This makes three sections – two small ones and one big one.

The big section is for vegetables, and the two smaller sections are for your starches and proteins. You can use this as a measuring guide when you go out to eat or want to transition your dinner plate into healthier portions.

You will receive the highest levels of phytonutrients from vegetables, so that is why vegetables occupy the largest section of the plate.

Eat slowly

It takes twenty minutes for your food to start digesting and give you a feeling of fullness when you eat your meals. Therefore, slow down and chew your foods so that you can actually taste and enjoy their flavors. If you tend to eat fast, you may find that you eat more because it takes that twenty minutes to get your internal system fired up.

Drink water before your meal

Try drinking a full eight-ounce glass of water before you sit down to eat a meal. Sometimes thirst can be mistaken for a feeling of hunger. Drinking a glass of water before you eat can get the digestion process started quicker which can cause you to eat less during a meal.

Exercise

Adhere to the lowest, most foundational level of the Mediterranean pyramid which is a daily activity. Do your best to get thirty minutes of exercise in every day.

Chapter 1: Mediterranean Appetizers Recipes

Sandwiches with Cheese, Salad, Olives, and Grapes

Prep time: 15 min | **Servings**: 12

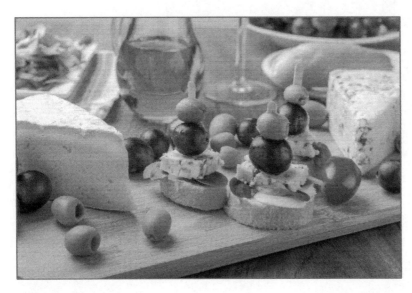

Nutritional Info (per serving):

- ✓ Calories – 112
- ✓ Fat – 4.3 g
- ✓ Fiber – 2.1 g
- ✓ Carbs – 12.9 g
- ✓ Protein – 5.9 g
- ✓ Sodium – 322 mg

A delicious way to start any occasion, an ideal appetizer which is very healthy and easy to prepare.

Ingredients:

- 12 slices of wheat bread
- 3 cups of fresh basil leaves
- 6 oz feta cheese, sliced or cubed
- 5 tbsp green olives
- 5 tbsp grapes
- 12 ice cream sticks

Directions:

1. Place the bread on a serving plate.
2. Put basil leaves and a piece of feta cheese on the bread.
3. Stab the ice cream stick into the center of the sandwich vertically.
4. Thread grapes and olives onto the stick.
5. Repeat the order for all the bread.
6. Serve and enjoy.

Stuffed Tomatoes

Prep time: 15 min | **Servings**: 12

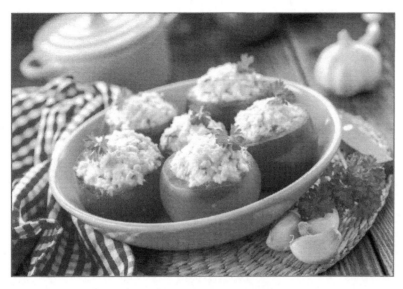

Nutritional Info (per serving):

- ✓ Calories – 154
- ✓ Fat – 10.4 g
- ✓ Fiber – 1.5 g
- ✓ Carbs – 8.1 g
- ✓ Protein – 9.2 g
- ✓ Sodium – 230 mg

A perfect Mediterranean appetizer for every occasion especially when you are enjoying with your friends and family.

Ingredients:

- 12 medium tomatoes

Stuffing:

- 2 oz cheese and garlic croutons
- 2 hard-boiled eggs, grated
- 12 tbsp Cheddar cheese, grated
- 12 tbsp Parmesan cheese, grated
- 2 cloves garlic, minced
- 2 tbsp olive oil
- 2 tbsp Greek yogurt
- ¼ cup fresh parsley, finely chopped
- ¼ tsp freshly ground pepper

Directions:

1. Cut the slices on the top of the tomatoes. Scoop out and set aside the pulp. Let tomatoes dry on a paper towel.
2. In a bowl mix all the ingredients to make a stuffing.
3. Stuff the tomatoes with the prepared stuffing.
4. Decorate stuffed tomatoes with parsley leaves.
5. Serve and enjoy!

Eggplant Rolls
Stuffed with Cream Cheese and Tomatoes

Prep time: 10 min | **Cooking time**: 6 min | **Servings**: 6

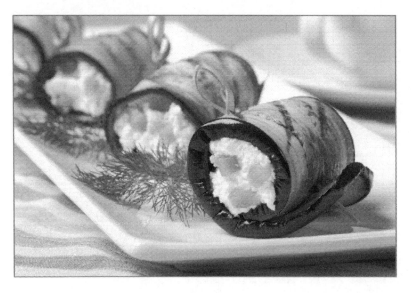

Nutritional Info (per serving):

- Calories – 91
- Fat – 7.0 g
- Fiber – 3.1 g
- Carbs – 6.3 g
- Protein – 2.1 g
- Sodium – 140 mg

This eggplant appetizer is easy to prepare and ideal for every family gatherings and friends who want to come over the weekend.

Ingredients:

- 1 large eggplant, ½ inch sliced lengthwise
- 1 tbsp olive oil
- ¼ tsp kosher salt
- ½ tsp ground black pepper
- ⅓ cup cream cheese
- ½ cup chopped tomatoes
- 1 clove garlic, minced
- 2 tbsp chopped dill

Directions:

1. On a plate, place the sliced eggplant, brush it with oil and season with salt and pepper.
2. Grill the eggplants on both sides for 3 minutes until golden brown.
3. In a separate bowl, combine the cream cheese, tomatoes, garlic and dill to form a mixture.
4. Cool down the eggplant slices and place 1 tbsp cream cheese mixture at the end of the eggplant slices and roll it over. Pin it with the toothpick to prevent it from unrolling.
5. Grease some oil and serve.

Mushrooms Stuffed with Cheese, Pepper, and Garlic

Prep time: 20 min | **Cooking time**: 25 min | **Servings**: 6

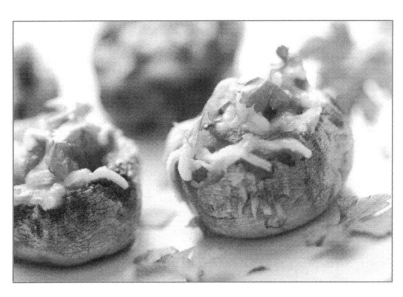

Nutritional Info (per serving):

- ✓ *Calories – 211*
- ✓ *Fat – 13.8 g*
- ✓ *Fiber – 1.0 g*
- ✓ *Carbs – 5.9 g*
- ✓ *Protein – 16.8 g*
- ✓ *Sodium – 361 mg*

A favorite dish for everybody, an easy to prepare and an instant crowd favorite.

Ingredients:

- 6 large Portabello mushrooms, stalks removed
- 8 tbsp grated Mozzarella cheese
- 18 tbsp grated Cheddar cheese
- 1 garlic clove, minced
- 1 tsp English mustard
- 1 tsp black pepper
- 1 white onion, finely chopped
- 1 large red sweet pepper, chopped

Directions:

1. Place the mushrooms bottom side up on a baking tray.
2. In a bowl, combine the mozzarella cheese, cheddar cheese, and garlic to form a mixture. Slowly add the mustard and black pepper to the mixture.
3. Finally, add the chopped onion and red sweet pepper to the mixture and mix it well.
4. Place the cheese mixture into the mushrooms and gently pat it.
5. Baked it in the 350°F oven over 25 minutes.
6. Serve and enjoy.

Greek Yogurt Dip

Prep time: 10 min | **Servings**: 4

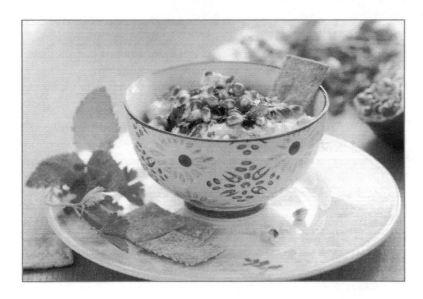

Nutritional Info (per serving):

- ✓ *Calories – 59*
- ✓ *Fat – 3.8 g*
- ✓ *Fiber – 0.4 g*
- ✓ *Carbs – 3.1 g*
- ✓ *Protein – 4.0 g*
- ✓ *Sodium – 183 mg*

A perfect dip to start every meal which makes your palate craves for a more sumptuous dish.

Ingredients:

- 1 cup Greek plain yogurt
- 1 tbsp fresh mint leaves, finely chopped
- 1 tbsp fresh dill, finely chopped
- 1 tbsp red onion, finely chopped
- 1 tbsp red wine vinegar
- ¼ tsp kosher salt
- 1 tbsp extra virgin olive oil
- 1 tbsp pomegranate seeds
- 1 tbsp olives, halved
- 1 sprig of parsley for decoration

Directions:

1. In a bowl combine yogurt, mint leaves, dill, red onion, kosher salt, vinegar, and olive oil and mix well.
2. Garnish with pomegranate seeds, olives, and parsley; then place it in the fridge before serving.

Chapter 2: Mediterranean Salads Recipes

Caprese Salad

Prep time: 15 min | **Servings**: 4

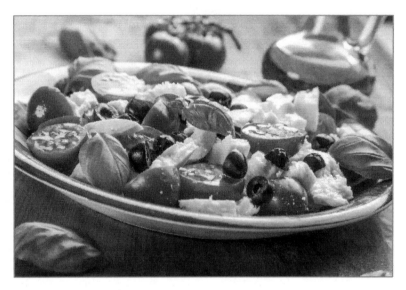

Nutritional Info (per serving):

- Calories – 118
- Fat – 9.1 g
- Fiber – 2.1 g
- Carbs – 7.7 g
- Protein – 3.6 g
- Sodium – 233 mg

A traditional Italian salad which is very easy to prepare.

Ingredients:

- 4 tomatoes, sliced
- 1 red pepper, chopped
- 2 tbsp black olives, sliced
- 1 cup Mozzarella cheese, cut into ¼-inch slices
- 1 cup basil leaves
- 2 tbsp olive oil
- ¼ tsp kosher salt

Directions:

1. In a serving plate combine basil leaves, tomatoes, red pepper, and mozzarella cheese.
2. Drizzle with olive oil, garnish with olives, and season with salt.
3. Bon Appetit!

Salad with Fresh Spinach, Tuna, and Feta Cheese

Prep time: 15 min | **Servings**: 4

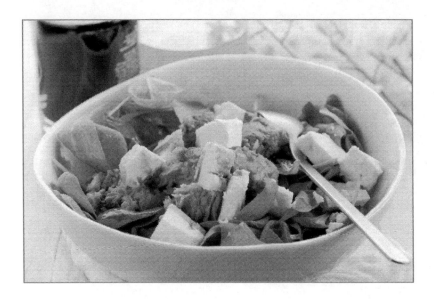

Nutritional Info (per serving):

- ✓ Calories – 206
- ✓ Fat – 11.1 g
- ✓ Fiber – 1.9 g
- ✓ Carbs – 3.8 g
- ✓ Protein – 23.6 g
- ✓ Sodium – 403 mg

This healthy salad ideal for people who are conscious about their cholesterol level. It is known that tuna have an omega-3 to lower bad cholesterol and reduce heart diseases.

Ingredients:

- 3 oz Tuna, chunked and cooked
- 3 oz fresh spinach leaves
- 2 oz feta cheese, sliced
- 2 tbsp olive oil
- ¼ tsp kosher salt
- ¼ tsp black pepper, freshly ground

Directions:

1. In a bowl, place the tuna, cut into serving pieces.
2. Wash and chop the leaves of spinach.
3. Add the spinach and feta cheese to the bowl with tuna.
4. Drizzle with olive oil. Season with salt and pepper to taste.
5. Serve and enjoy.

Fresh Green Salad with Shrimps and Avocado

Prep time: 15 min | **Servings**: 8

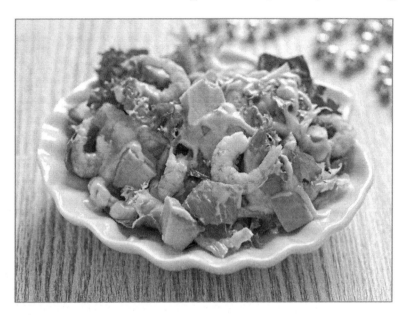

Nutritional Info (per serving):

- Calories – 133
- Fat – 11.0 g
- Fiber – 2.8 g
- Carbs – 9.1 g
- Protein – 4.5 g
- Sodium – 244 mg

A sumptuous salad ideal for every occasion and events which makes everyone lightens and refresh.

Ingredients:

- 5 cups mixed baby greens
- 3 oz avocado, cut into cubes
- 3 oz shrimps, cooked and peeled
- 5 tbsp extra virgin olive oil
- ¼ tsp paprika
- 1 tsp Dijon mustard
- 1 ½ tbsp wine vinegar
- ¼ tsp black pepper, freshly ground
- ½ tsp salt

Directions:

1. In a bowl combine the mixed baby greens, avocado, and shrimps.
2. In a separate bowl mix the paprika, olive oil, Dijon mustard, and vinegar to make a dressing.
3. Pour the dressing over the salad and season with salt and pepper to taste.
4. Serve and enjoy.

Salad with Fish and Fresh Vegetables

Prep time: 15 min | **Servings**: 6

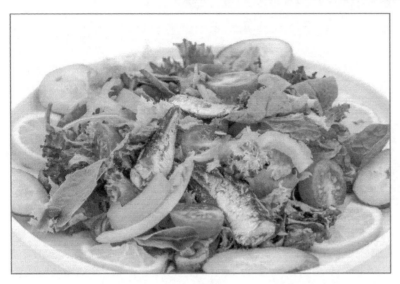

Nutritional Info (per serving):

- Calories – 120
- Fat – 6.9 g
- Fiber – 3.2 g
- Carbs – 15.9 g
- Protein – 5.8 g
- Sodium – 313 mg

A classic Mediterranean salad is healthy and easy to prepare. Fish are rich in essential oils and nutrients needed to lower the risk of heart diseases. This salad is perfect with friends catching up over a weekend.

Ingredients:

- 3 oz sardines, steamed and head removed
- 1 cucumber, sliced
- 1 yellow bell pepper, sliced
- 2 cups spinach, chopped
- 1 cup lettuce, shredded and chopped
- 4 tomatoes, sliced
- 1 onion, sliced
- 2 small lemons, sliced
- 1 cup basil leaves
- 1 tsp mustard
- 2 tbsp olive oil
- 1 ½ tbsp wine vinegar
- 1 tsp black pepper, freshly ground
- ½ tsp kosher salt

Directions:

1. In a bowl toss the fish, cucumber, yellow bell pepper, spinach, lettuce, tomatoes, onion, lemons, and basil leaves.
2. In a separate bowl mix olive oil, mustard, and vinegar to make a dressing.
3. Pour the dressing over the salad and season with salt and pepper to taste.
4. Serve and enjoy.

Red Beans and Greens Salad

Prep time: 10 min | **Servings**: 6

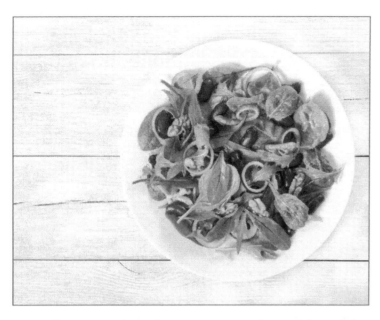

Nutritional Info (per serving):

- ✓ *Calories – 242*
- ✓ *Fat – 13.7 g*
- ✓ *Fiber – 6.2 g*
- ✓ *Carbs – 22.7 g*
- ✓ *Protein – 10.1 g*
- ✓ *Sodium – 121 mg*

A perfect appetizer for every occasion with red beans; it will surely make your event a memorable one.

Ingredients:

- 1 cup organic red beans, cooked and drained
- 1 cup lettuce, shredded and chopped
- 2 cups spinach leaves
- ½ cup walnut, halved
- 1 cup red onion, cut into thin rings
- 3 tbsp fresh lemon juice
- 3 tbsp extra virgin olive oil
- 1 tsp Dijon mustard
- 1 clove of garlic, minced
- ¼ tsp salt
- ¼ tsp freshly ground pepper

Directions:

1. In a bowl combine the red beans, lettuce, spinach, walnut and red onion.
2. In a separate bowl mix the lemon juice, olive oil, garlic and Dijon mustard to make a dressing.
3. Pour the dressing over the salad and season with salt and pepper to taste.
4. Serve and enjoy.

Bulgur Salad

Prep time: 10 min | **Cooking time**: 20 min | **Servings**: 6

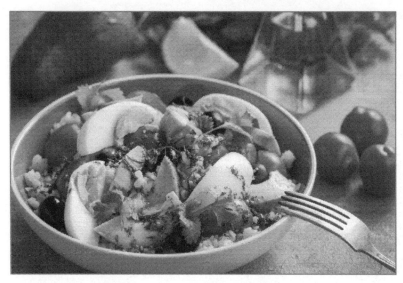

Nutritional Info (per serving):

- Calories – 326
- Fat – 16.5 g
- Fiber – 11.5 g
- Carbs – 40.6 g
- Protein – 8.8 g
- Sodium – 249 mg

A classic Mediterranean salad perfect for guest and friends who loved to lose weight without sacrificing their appetite.

Ingredients:

- 2 cups bulgur
- 4 cups water
- 1 tbsp butter, unsalted
- 2 tbsp olive oil
- 1 medium avocado, chopped
- ¼ cup dill, chopped
- 2 tsp red wine vinegar
- 8 tbsp olives, pitted and chopped
- 2 hard-boiled eggs, sliced
- ½ cup tomato cherries
- ¼ tsp salt

Directions:

1. Place a saucepan over medium heat and add 1 tbsp of butter and 1 tbsp of olive oil. Toast the bulgur in the oil until it turns golden brown and starts to crackle.
2. Add 4 cups of water to the saucepan and season with the salt. Cover the saucepan and simmer until all the water gets absorbed for about 20 minutes.
3. Allow the bulgur to cool and transfer it into the serving dishes.
4. In a mixing bowl, combine the chopped avocado with eggs, tomatoes, dill, olives, red wine vinegar and the remaining olive oil.
5. Serve this over the bulgur.
6. Garnish with parsley.

Colorful Vegetable Salad

Prep time: 10 min | **Servings**: 8

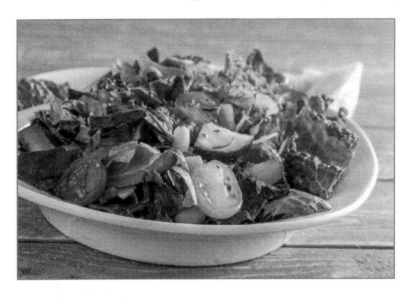

Nutritional Info (per serving):

- ✓ *Calories* – 125
- ✓ *Fat* – 9.4 g
- ✓ *Fiber* – 1.4 g
- ✓ *Carbs* – 9.1 g
- ✓ *Protein* – 3.0 g
- ✓ *Sodium* – 315 mg

A delicious salad easy to prepare and healthy for everyone.

Ingredients:

- 2 cups kale, chopped
- 2 cups lettuce, shredded and chopped
- 1 ½ cups cucumber, diced
- 1 cup cherry tomatoes, quartered
- ½ cup olives
- ½ cup Feta cheese, crumbled
- 1 red or yellow peppers, diced
- 1 lemon juice
- 1 tbsp honey
- ¼ cup extra virgin olive oil
- 2 tsp oregano leaves, dried
- ½ tsp salt
- ½ tsp black pepper, freshly ground

Directions:

1. In a bowl toss together the kale, lettuce, cucumber, tomatoes, olives, feta cheese, red or yellow peppers.
2. In a separate bowl, combine the lemon juice, honey, olive oil and dried oregano leaves. Add salt and pepper to taste.
3. Drizzle the dressing over the salad. Serve and enjoy.

Chapter 3: Mediterranean Vegetable Recipes

Sautéed Greek Zucchini

Prep time: 7 min | **Cooking time**: 15 min | **Servings**: 2

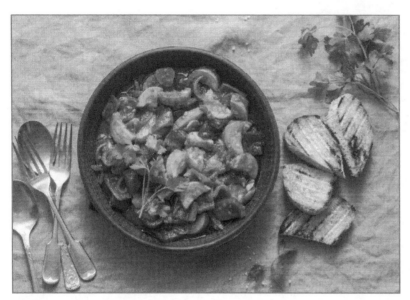

Nutritional Info (per serving):
- Calories – 205
- Fat – 14.6 g
- Fiber – 4.3 g
- Carbs – 19.1 g
- Protein – 3.4 g
- Sodium – 252 mg

This simple Mediterranean vegetable dish is ideal for unexpected guests.

Ingredients:
- 2 tbsp olive oil
- 2 small zucchini, cut into pieces
- 1 medium red onion, chopped
- 1 red bell pepper, cut into strips
- 1 green bell pepper, cut into strips
- 2 tsp Greek seasonings
- 2 tsp balsamic vinegar
- ½ tsp garlic, minced
- ⅛ tsp salt
- ½ tsp sugar

Directions:
1. In a medium heat pan, sauté the zucchini, onion, red and green pepper in 2 tbsp olive oil.
2. In a small bowl, mix 1 tbsp olive oil, Greek seasonings, balsamic vinegar, garlic, salt, and sugar to make a sauce.
3. Pour the sauce over the vegetables until fully coated.
4. Garnish with parsley. Serve and enjoy.

Stuffed Eggplant with Fried Vegetables

Prep time: 13 min | **Cooking time**: 30 min | **Servings**: 2

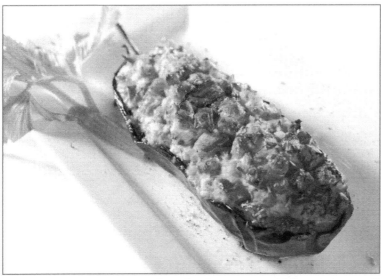

Nutritional Info (per serving):

- ✓ Calories – 385
- ✓ Fat – 18.4 g
- ✓ Fiber – 21.0 g
- ✓ Carbs – 51.0 g
- ✓ Protein – 15.6 g
- ✓ Sodium – 372 mg

A perfect dish for people who love vegetables, an eggplant with stuffing is a twist that your family will surely love.

Ingredients:

- 1 medium eggplant
- 1 onion, chopped
- 1 green pepper, chopped
- 2 stalks celery, chopped
- 2 large leeks, chopped
- 1 tbsp olive oil
- 2 tbsp fresh thyme
- 1 tbsp chives
- 1 tbsp parsley
- 2 fresh tomatoes, chopped
- ½ cup wheat bran
- ⅛ tsp salt
- ¼ tsp black pepper, freshly ground
- 2 oz Cheddar cheese, grated

Directions:

1. Cut the eggplant into lengthwise halves. Scoop out the pulp and chopped into pieces. Set aside.
2. In a medium heat pan, sauté eggplant pulp in the olive oil. Add chopped onion, pepper, celery, and leeks and cook until tender.
3. Add the thyme, chives, parsley, tomatoes, wheat bran, salt, and pepper and mix well.
4. Place the eggplant on a baking pan and stuff it with the prepared stuffing.
5. Bake the eggplant at 400°F for 30 min.
6. 10 minutes before the end of cooking sprinkle top with Cheddar cheese.
7. Garnish with fresh celery. Serve and enjoy.

Vegetarian Mushroom Casserole

Prep time: 13 min | **Cooking time**: 30 min | **Servings**: 4

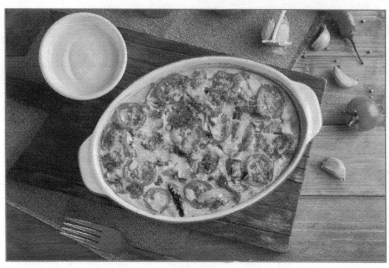

Nutritional Info (per serving):

- Calories – 187
- Fat – 11.0 g
- Fiber – 4.1 g
- Carbs – 16.1 g
- Protein – 8.9 g
- Sodium – 425 mg

In this casserole, vegetables and mushrooms perfectly complement each other. Enjoy this easy-to-prepare and delicate dish!

Ingredients:

- 2 cup broccoli
- 1 cup cauliflower
- 1 red pepper, chopped
- 1 carrot, finely chopped
- 1 onion, finely chopped
- 1 clove garlic, minced
- 1 cup mushrooms, cooked and cut into halves
- ½ tsp kosher salt
- ¼ tsp black pepper, freshly ground
- 2 medium tomatoes, sliced into rings
- 2/3 cup sour cream
- 2 oz Mozzarella cheese, shredded
- 1 tbsp parsley to garnish

Directions:

1. In a large bowl, mix broccoli, cauliflower, pepper, carrot, onion, garlic, and mushrooms. Season with salt and pepper.
2. Transfer the mixture to the baking pan and put sliced tomatoes on top.
3. Pour the sour cream and sprinkle with shredded cheese on top.
4. Bake casserole at 350°F for 30 minutes.
5. Garnish with parsley. Serve and enjoy.

Moroccan Style Vegetable Stew

Prep time: 13 min | **Cooking time**: 30 min | **Servings**: 6

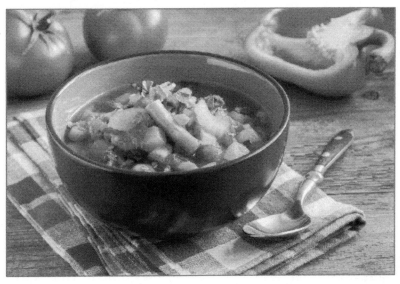

Nutritional Info (per serving):

- ✓ *Calories – 179*
- ✓ *Fat – 5.3 g*
- ✓ *Fiber – 6.3 g*
- ✓ *Carbs – 31.4 g*
- ✓ *Protein – 4.0 g*
- ✓ *Sodium – 130mg*

A delicious stew with beans and potatoes in a Moroccan style is perfect for everyone.

Ingredients:

- 2 tbsp olive oil
- 1 garlic clove, finely chopped
- 2 large onions, finely chopped
- 2 large carrots, chopped
- 2 bell peppers, chopped
- 4 medium tomatoes, diced
- 3 medium potatoes, cubed
- ½ cup green beans, chopped
- 1 cup water
- 2 tsp ground cumin
- ½ tsp ground turmeric
- 1 tsp dried hot red pepper flakes
- ¼ tsp kosher salt
- ¼ tsp black pepper, freshly ground
- 2 tsp fresh coriander leaves, chopped to garnish

Directions:

1. In a medium-heat pan pour olive oil and sauté garlic with onions until golden brown.
2. Add carrots, peppers, and tomatoes, and sauté for 5 minutes.
3. Add potatoes with green beans and sauté another 5 minutes.
4. Pour the water, bring to a boil and simmer for 20 minutes until vegetables are tender.
5. Season with cumin, turmeric, red pepper flakes, salt and black pepper.
6. Garnish with chopped coriander. Serve and enjoy.

Mediterranean Chickpea Patties

Prep time: 10 min | **Cooking time**: 15 min | **Servings**: 8

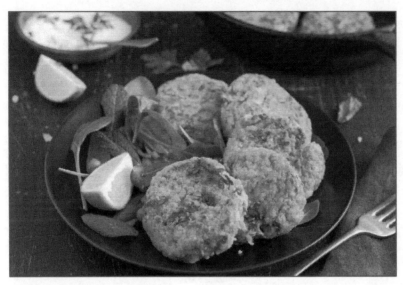

Nutritional Info (per serving):

- ✓ Calories – 352
- ✓ Fat – 27.1 g
- ✓ Fiber – 3.8 g
- ✓ Carbs – 24.0 g
- ✓ Protein – 6.1 g
- ✓ Sodium – 166mg

These delicious chickpea patties can be served with a sauce or greens for a Mediterranean breakfast or dinner.

Ingredients:

- 1 cup flour
- ½ tsp salt
- ½ tsp ground cumin
- 1 egg, whisked
- ¾ cup hot water
- 1 cup chopped fresh spinach
- 3 garlic cloves, minced
- ⅛ tsp baking soda
- ¾ cup chickpeas, cooked
- 2 small chopped scallions
- 1 cup extra-virgin olive oil

Directions:

1. In a large bowl mix together the flour, salt, and cumin. Add egg, and the water to make a batter. Whisk thoroughly until thickened.
2. Stir the spinach, garlic, baking soda, chickpeas and scallions into the batter. Mix until well blended.
3. In a high heat pan, add the olive oil until simmering. Pour one tablespoon of batter into the oil and deep fry it on both sides.
4. Repeat until all batter is used.
5. First, place the fried frittata on a paper towel, and then transfer it to a serving plate.
6. Garnish with greens and lime and enjoy.

Braised Leeks

Prep time: 5 min | **Cooking time**: 20 min | **Servings**: 3

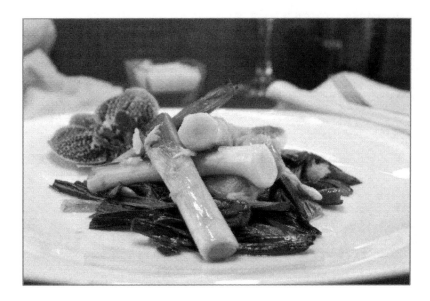

Nutritional Info (per serving):

- ✓ *Calories – 242*
- ✓ *Fat – 17.5 g*
- ✓ *Fiber – 1.7 g*
- ✓ *Carbs – 14.0 g*
- ✓ *Protein – 2.3 g*
- ✓ *Sodium – 368 mg*

Leek is rich in vitamins and microelements, such as phosphorus and magnesium. Also, leek contains a large number of coarse fibers, which cause intestinal motility to work actively.

Ingredients:

- 3 leeks, trimmed and cut into halves
- 2 tbsp unsalted butter
- 2 tbsp olive oil
- ½ cup broth
- ½ cup white wine
- 1 tsp fresh thyme, finely chopped
- ¼ tsp salt
- ⅛ tsp black pepper, freshly ground

Directions:

1. Clean the leeks trimmed the outer leaves. Cut the leeks into halves.
2. In a medium heat pan, melt the butter with oil. Place the leeks and stir it for 5 minutes.
3. Add broth, wine, and thyme and let it simmer for 15 minutes.
4. Season with salt and pepper.
5. Serve and enjoy.

Chapter 4: Mediterranean Seafood Recipes

Salmon Skewers with Pepper and Spices

Prep time: 15 min | **Cooking time**: 16 min | **Servings**: 4

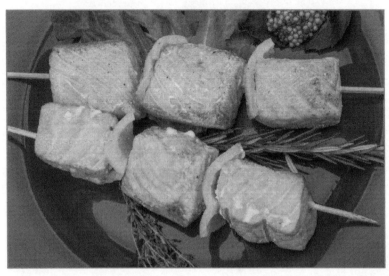

Nutritional Info (per serving):
- Calories – 172
- Fat – 7.2 g
- Fiber – 0.7 g
- Carbs – 5.1 g
- Protein – 22.3 g
- Sodium – 189 mg

A perfect picnic dish for a family gathering and for simple occasions like catching up with friends over the weekend.

Ingredients:
- 1 lbs salmon fillet, cubed
- 1 lemon juice
- 1 tsp dried thyme
- 1 tsp dried rosemary
- ¼ tsp salt
- ¼ tsp freshly ground black pepper
- 1 green bell pepper, sliced

Directions:
1. Season the salmon with lemon juice, thyme, rosemary, salt, and pepper.
2. Slide the salmon onto the skewers with green pepper alternately.
3. Grill the skewed salmon over the medium heat for 16 minutes turning the sides every 4 minutes.
4. Transfer the cooked salmon to the serving plate.
5. Serve with fresh herbs and enjoy.

Baked Salmon with Vegetables Ratatouille

Prep time: 13 min | **Cooking time**: 1 hour 12 min | **Servings**: 4

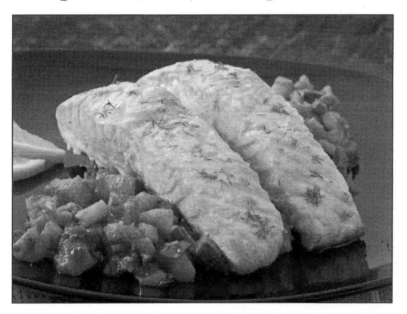

Nutritional Info (per serving):

- ✓ Calories – 339
- ✓ Fat – 15.0 g
- ✓ Fiber – 6.3 g
- ✓ Carbs – 17.1 g
- ✓ Protein – 37.1 g
- ✓ Sodium – 376 mg

Ingredients:

- 1 red onion, roughly chopped
- 2 cloves garlic, chopped
- 1 tbsp olive oil
- 1 eggplant, cubed
- 1 medium green zucchini, cut into about 1-inch pieces
- 1 cup ripe tomatoes, chopped
- ½ tsp paprika
- 1 tbsp water
- 2 salmon fillets
- 1 cup red pepper, chopped
- 1 lemon zest and juice
- 2 tbsp fresh basil
- ½ tsp kosher salt
- ¼ tsp freshly ground pepper

Directions:

1. In a baking dish, toss the onion, garlic and olive oil until coated.
2. Add the eggplant, zucchini, tomatoes, paprika, and water. Mix well to combine.
3. Cover baking dish with the foil. Bake at 340°F for 1 hour.
4. In a bowl, combine the salmon with lemon zest and juice to marinate. Place marinated salmon on the top of the ratatouille. Take the red peppers and toss to coat. Return the baking dish back to the oven and bake salmon with vegetables for another 12-14 minutes.
5. When it is ready, remove from the oven and garnish with basil over the top. Season with salt and pepper to taste.
6. Serve and enjoy.

Salmon Steak Fillet with Cheese Crust Breading

Prep time: 12 min | **Cooking time**: 25 min | **Servings**: 2

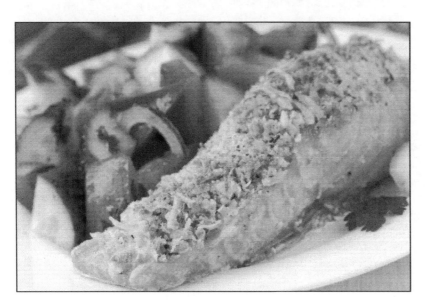

Nutritional Info (per serving):

- ✓ Calories – 323
- ✓ Fat – 16.7 g
- ✓ Fiber – 1.2 g
- ✓ Carbs – 14.9 g
- ✓ Protein – 29.1 g
- ✓ Sodium – 456mg

A delicious dish for everyone and easy to prepare.

Ingredients:

- 2 salmon fillets
- 1 tbsp butter, melted
- ⅛ tsp salt
- ⅓ cup fresh white breadcrumbs
- 1 oz Parmesan cheese, grated
- 2 tbsp onion, finely chopped
- 2 tsp lemon peel, grated
- ¼ tsp dried thyme leaves

Directions:

1. In a bowl mix melted butter, salt, breadcrumbs, cheese, onion, lemon peel, and thyme to make a coating.
2. Dredge the salmon in the cheese coating until evenly coated and place it in the baking dish.
3. Bake it at 375°F for 25 minutes.
4. Best serve with vegetable salad and enjoy.

Crispy Grilled Salmon Steak

Prep time: 5 min | **Cooking time**: 20 min | **Servings**: 2

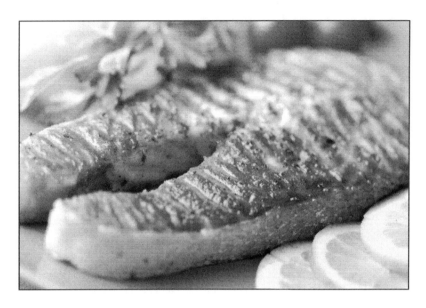

Nutritional Info (per serving):

- *Calories – 354*
- *Fat – 18.9 g*
- *Fiber – 2.2 g*
- *Carbs – 12.4 g*
- *Protein – 35.8 g*
- *Sodium – 372 mg*

A crispy grilled salmon perfect for salmon lovers, an ideal for every occasion and a sure crowd favorite.

Ingredients:

- 2 salmon steak
- 1 tbsp unsalted butter
- 1 tsp olive oil
- 1 tsp thyme, dried
- 1 lemon juice
- ¼ tsp salt
- ¼ tsp freshly ground black pepper
- ¼ cup wheat flour, whole-grain

Directions:

1. In a bowl, combine the butter, olive oil, thyme, and lemon juice to make a dip.
2. Season the salmon with salt and black pepper.
3. Dip the salmon into butter mixture and coat on both sides with flour.
4. Grill the salmon for 20 minutes, for 10 minutes each side.
5. Serve with lemon slices and enjoy.

Grilled Tuna Steak with Red Wine Sauce

Prep time: 5 min | **Cooking time:** 20 min | **Servings:** 4

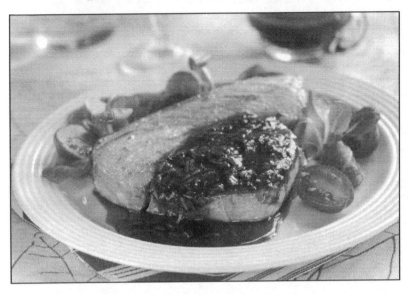

Nutritional Info (per serving):

- Calories – 461
- Fat – 23.5 g
- Fiber – 0.2 g
- Carbs – 4.1 g
- Protein – 51.0 g
- Sodium – 398 mg

Tuna is valuable fish. In tuna meat there are no carbohydrates, this product is low-calorie. Tuna meat contains a huge amount of nutrients, such as polyunsaturated fatty acids omega-3 and omega-6 and some microelements. Systematic eating of this fish reduces the risk of cardiovascular disease by about half. Now you can enjoy a delicious dish at the comfort of your home like in a fine seafood dining.

Ingredients:

- 4 tuna steak, above 6-oz and 1-inch thick
- 2 tsp thyme, dried
- ½ tsp salt
- ¼ tsp freshly ground black pepper
- 2 tbsp olive oil

For Sauce:

- 2 tsp honey
- 2 tbsp unsalted butter
- ½ cup red wine
- 1 tsp fresh parsley, finely chopped

Directions:

1. Season the tuna with thyme, salt, and black pepper.
2. In a medium-high heat, sear the salmon in the olive oil until golden brown on both sides. Set aside.
3. In a bowl, whisk the honey with butter until well blended. Add the red wine and continue to whisk.
4. In low heat, simmer the sauce until reduced by about half. At the end of cooking add parsley.
5. Pour the sauce over the tuna steak. Serve and enjoy.

Grilled Sea Bass with Parsley and Lemon

Prep time: 8 min | **Cooking time**: 22 min | **Servings**: 4

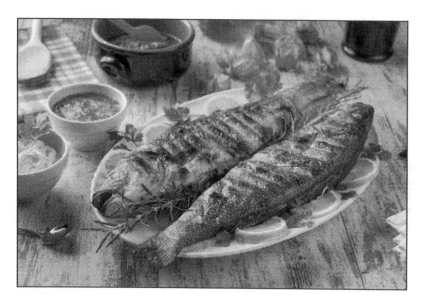

Nutritional Info (per serving):

- Calories – 296
- Fat – 6.7 g
- Fiber – 1.8 g
- Carbs – 29.1 g
- Protein – 29.5 g
- Sodium – 478mg

A perfect picnic recipe that will make your family and friends meeting memorable.

Ingredients:

- 2 whole sea bass, about 1 lbs each
- ¾ tsp salt
- ½ tsp freshly ground black pepper
- 1 tsp fresh parsley, chopped
- 1 tsp fresh thyme, chopped
- 1 lemon, wedged

Directions:

1. Clean the sea bass. Wash it thoroughly. Pat it dry with paper towel.
2. Season with salt, black pepper, parsley, and thyme.
3. Grill sea bass for 12 minutes or until skin golden brown. Then turn over and grill another 10 minutes until cooked.
4. Serve with herbs and lemon wedges.

Shrimps and Vegetables Stir-Fry

Prep time: 10 min | **Cooking time**: 17 min | **Servings**: 4

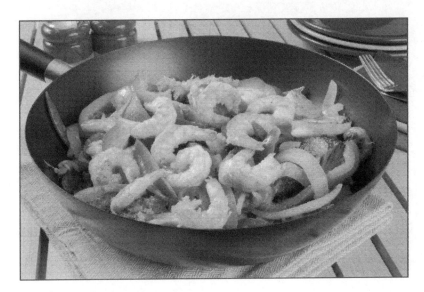

Nutritional Info (per serving):

- ✓ Calories – 154
- ✓ Fat – 7.9 g
- ✓ Fiber – 3.4 g
- ✓ Carbs – 13.2 g
- ✓ Protein – 9.5 g
- ✓ Sodium – 372 mg

Ingredients:

- 4 oz shrimps, peeled
- 2 tbsp olive oil
- 1 large onion, cut into rings
- 1 cloves garlic, minced
- 1 red bell pepper, cut into strips
- 1 green bell pepper, cut into strips
- 1 cup broccoli florets
- 1 cup snow peas
- ½ tsp salt
- ½ tsp red pepper flakes
- ⅛ tsp ground ginger

Directions:

1. Wash the shrimps under the cold water. Set aside.
2. Cook broccoli in boiling water for 5-7 minutes. Drain the water and set aside.
3. In a medium-high heat pan, sauté the onion and the garlic in olive oil.
4. Once the onion became translucent, add bell peppers, broccoli, and the snow peas. Stir for 7-10 minutes or until tender over medium-high heat.
5. Add the shrimps and stir for 3-5 minutes until pink.
6. Season with salt, red pepper flakes, and ground ginger.
7. Serve and enjoy.

Shrimps with Asparagus, Tomatoes, and Paprika

Prep time: 15min | **Cooking time**: 30 min | **Servings**: 4

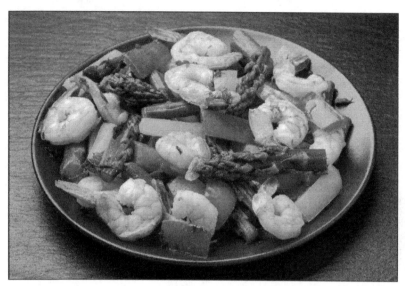

Nutritional Info (per serving):

- Calories – 174
- Fat – 11.4 g
- Fiber – 2.7 g
- Carbs – 11.4 g
- Protein – 8.7 g
- Sodium – 516 mg

Delicious and easy to prepare shrimp recipe that your friends and family will always love.

Ingredients:

- 4 oz raw shrimp
- 3 tbsp olive oil
- 1 large onion, finely chopped
- 1 clove garlic, minced
- 1 ripe tomato, chopped
- 1 red bell pepper, cut into strips
- 1 yellow bell pepper, cut into strips
- 4 oz asparagus
- 1 tsp paprika
- ½ tsp kosher salt
- ½ tsp ground ginger
- 1 tbsp low sodium soy sauce
- 2 tbsp lemon juice

Directions:

1. Peel and wash the shrimps under the cold water.
2. In a medium-high heat pan, stir shrimps in 2 tablespoons olive oil for 5 minutes until pink. Then remove shrimps from the pan and set aside.
3. In the same pan, sauté the onion and the garlic in remaining olive oil.
4. Add the tomatoes, peppers and asparagus and stew 20 minutes until tender.
5. Return the shrimps and season with paprika, salt, ground ginger, and soy sauce.
6. Mix well, add lemon juice and stir for 1-2 minutes.
7. Serve and enjoy.

BAKED SALMON WITH LEMON AND CHERRY TOMATOES

Prep time: 8 min | **Cooking time**: 25 min | **Servings**: 4

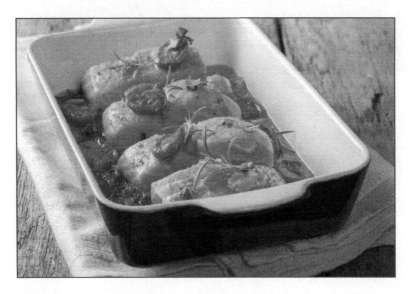

Nutritional Info (per serving):

- ✓ Calories – 346
- ✓ Fat – 21.8 g
- ✓ Fiber – 1.2 g
- ✓ Carbs – 4.1 g
- ✓ Protein – 35.5 g
- ✓ Sodium – 233mg

Salmon is always the healthier choice for people who love to be fit, with this recipe your guest will surely love salmon like never before. Moreover, this dish is the Keto-friendly.

Ingredients:

- 4 salmon fillets, 6-oz each
- ¼ tsp salt
- ¼ tsp freshly ground black pepper
- 2 tbsp lemon juice
- 3 tbsp olive oil, extra virgin
- 2 cups cherry tomatoes, sliced in halves
- 1 clove garlic, minced
- rosemary leaves to garnish

Directions:

1. Preheat the oven to 420°F.
2. Season salmon fillets with salt, black pepper, and lemon juice.
3. Pour olive oil and arrange salmon fillets into the baking dish.
4. Sprinkle the remaining ingredients over the fillets.
5. Bake in the oven for 25 minutes or until salmon can easily be flaked.
6. Serve with fresh rosemary leaves and enjoy.

Roasted Garlic Butter Salmon

Prep time: 8 min | **Cooking time**: 20 min | **Servings**: 8

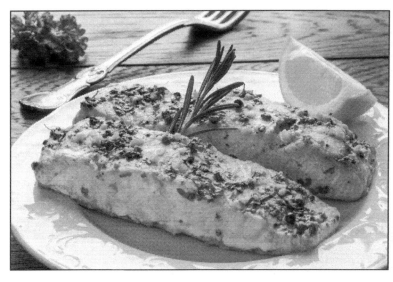

Nutritional Info (per serving):

- ✓ Calories – 294
- ✓ Fat – 17.4 g
- ✓ Fiber – 0.1 g
- ✓ Carbs – 0.5 g
- ✓ Protein – 34.7 g
- ✓ Sodium – 247mg

A beautiful dish ideal for every occasion, a sure crowd pleaser and a perfect salmon for everyone.

Ingredients:

- 8 salmon fillets, 6-oz each
- 2 tbsp extra virgin olive oil
- 2 tbsp lemon juice
- ½ tsp salt
- 2 tbsp butter, melted
- 2 cloves garlic
- 1 tsp peppercorns
- 1 tbsp chopped basil
- 1 tsp chopped parsley

Directions:

1. Preheat the oven to 350°F.
2. Place salmon fillets on the baking dish and brush each side with olive oil. Make sure that the skin side is facing down. Season with salt.
3. Pour the remaining olive oil and the lemon juice all over the fillets.
4. In a bowl, combine melted butter, garlic, and peppercorns; then pour mixture over the fillets. Sprinkle the basil and the parsley on the top of the fillets.
5. Let fillets bake in the oven for 20 minutes or until salmon can be easily flaked.

Chapter 5: Mediterranean Grains and Legumes Recipes

Garbanzos Greek Hummus

Prep time: 3 min | **Cooking time**: 5 min | **Servings**: 6

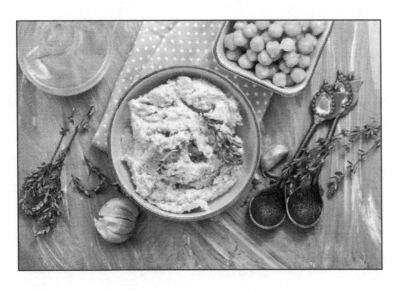

Nutritional Info (per serving):

- Calories – 206
- Fat – 9.5 g
- Fiber – 6.7 g
- Carbs – 23.8 g
- Protein – 8.2 g
- Sodium – 206 mg

A dish that will start your day full of energy and it is easy to prepare.

Ingredients:

- 3 cups garbanzo beans, boiled and drained
- 1 clove garlic, minced
- 2 tbsp lemon juice
- 2 tbsp tahini
- ½ tsp salt
- 2 tbsp olive oil, extra virgin
- fresh ground black pepper to taste

Directions:

1. Add the garbanzo beans, garlic, lemon juice, tahini, salt, and olive oil in a blender and blend until smooth.
2. Pour mixture into a serving bowl.
3. Drizzle some olive oil and sprinkle some ground black pepper on top.
4. Serve and decorate with herbs.

Oatmeal with Strawberry

Prep time: 10 min | **Cooking time**: 1 hour 10 min | **Servings**: 4

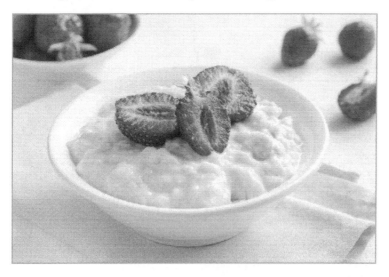

Nutritional Info (per serving):

- ✓ Calories – 135
- ✓ Fat – 4.3 g
- ✓ Fiber – 1.7 g
- ✓ Carbs – 19.1 g
- ✓ Protein – 5.6 g
- ✓ Sodium – 204 mg

Groats from whole grains are cooked longer than from ground or crushed grains. But they are used in the Mediterranean diet because of their health benefits. Whole grain oat is rich in B vitamins and magnesium. Oatmeal with Strawberry is delicious breakfast that your family will surely love.

Ingredients:

- 1 cup whole oat groats
- 1 ¼ cup water
- 1 ¾ cup milk
- ¼ tsp salt
- 2 tbsp sour cream
- 3 oz strawberry, thinly sliced or halved
- 2 tbsp brown sugar

Directions:

1. In the saucepan, bring whole oat groats and water to a boil. Cover and simmer on low for 30 minutes.
2. Add the milk and salt. Return to a boil and simmer for 20 to 30 minutes until creamy.
3. Uncover and simmer an additional 5-10 minutes occasionally stirring until desired consistency.
4. Remove from heat and let stand for 10 minutes.
5. Add the sour cream and stir well.
6. At that time toss the strawberry with the sugar in a bowl.
7. Transfer oatmeal to the serving bowls and top with strawberry mixture.
8. Serve and enjoy.

Baked Beans

Prep time: 2 hours 30 min | **Cooking time**: 50 min | **Servings**: 4

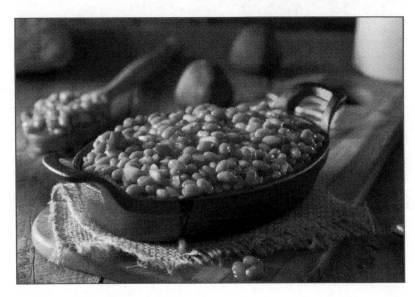

Nutritional Info (per serving):

- Calories – 183
- Fat – 4.3 g
- Fiber – 7.6 g
- Carbs – 26.2 g
- Protein – 11.3 g
- Sodium – 466mg

An ideal dish for everyone especially who have a steady day ahead.

Ingredients:

- 4 oz dry beans
- 1 onion, finely chopped
- 1 red bell pepper, finely chopped
- ¼ cup brown sugar
- ¼ tsp kosher salt
- ¼ tsp ground black pepper
- 1/3 cup ketchup
- 1 tbsp yellow mustard
- ½ tsp Worcestershire sauce (optional)
- ¼ tsp liquid smoke
- ¼ cup water

Directions:

1. First, soak the beans for 30 minutes in a bowl, then transfer it to a boiling pan and simmer on low for 2 hours.
2. Drain the beans. Place it in a large bowl along with the other ingredients and stir until well mixed.
3. Transfer the beans mixture to a baking dish, cover with a foil and bake at 350°F for 50 minutes to one hour.
4. Remove from the oven. Serve and enjoy.

Seafood Paella

Prep time: 5 min | **Cooking time**: 30 min | **Servings**: 8

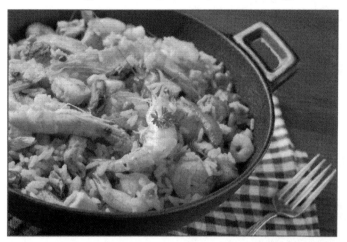

Nutritional Info (per serving):

- ✓ Calories – 351
- ✓ Fat – 5.4 g
- ✓ Fiber – 3.4 g
- ✓ Carbs – 46.6 g
- ✓ Protein – 27.5 g
- ✓ Sodium – 553 mg

Ingredients:

- 1 lobster tail, approx 4-oz weight
- 3 ½ cups water, divided
- 2 tbsp extra virgin olive oil
- 1 large yellow onion, chopped
- 4 garlic cloves, chopped
- 2 cups long grain rice, soaked in water for 15 minutes and then drained
- 2 tsp saffron soaked in ½ cup of water for yellow coloring
- 1 tsp paprika
- 1 tsp cayenne pepper
- ½ tsp ground black pepper
- ½ tsp salt
- 2 large tomatoes, finely chopped
- 6 oz fresh green beans, trimmed
- 1 lbs prawns, peeled and deveined
- ¼ cup chopped fresh parsley

Directions:

1. In a medium high heat pan, boil 2 cups of water. Put the lobster tail in the boiling water.
2. Let it simmer for 2 minutes until cooked. Then remove lobster from the water, let it a little cool down, remove the skins and chop. Set aside the broth for later use.
3. In a medium high heat pan, heat the olive oil and sauté the onion and garlic.
4. Add the rice and cook for 1 to 2 minutes. Keep mixing all the time.
5. Add the remaining water and the saffron soaked in water and the lobster broth. Cover the pan and simmer on low for 10 minutes.
6. Add the paprika, cayenne pepper, ground black pepper, salt, tomatoes, and green beans. Stir well, cover the pan and let it simmer for 10 minutes.
7. If need, uncover and allow excess liquid to evaporate for 1 to 2 minutes, stirring often.
8. Add the prawns over the rice and cook it for another 3 minutes.
9. Add the lobster tails and sprinkle the parsley. Serve and enjoy.

Quinoa Heaven

Prep time: 3 min | **Cooking time**: 15 min | **Servings**: 5

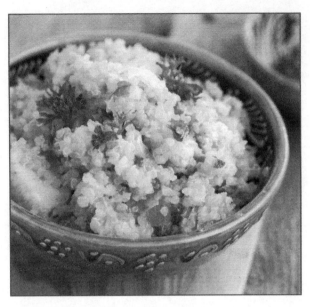

Nutritional Info (per serving):

- ✓ Calories – 344
- ✓ Fat – 13.8 g
- ✓ Fiber – 6.1 g
- ✓ Carbs – 45.7 g
- ✓ Protein – 12.6 g
- ✓ Sodium – 96 mg

Enjoy this feeling meal that is going to touch your taste buds in all the right ways as well as nourish your body with essential nutrients.

Ingredients:

- 1 cup almonds
- 1 cup quinoa
- 1 tsp cinnamon, ground
- 2 cups milk
- 1 tsp vanilla extract
- 1 pinch sea salt
- 2 tbsp honey
- 3 dates, dried, pitted and finely chopped
- 5 apricots, dried and finely chopped

Directions:

1. Start by toasting almonds in a skillet for five minutes or until golden brown for perfect nutty flavor. Set aside.
2. Put quinoa and cinnamon into a saucepan and place it over medium heat until warmed through. Follow by adding the milk, vanilla extract, and sea salt while stirring all along. Once the mixture comes to a boil, reduce the heat and cover the saucepan and let it simmer for 15 minutes.
3. Add the honey, dates, apricots, and half the almonds into the saucepan and stir well.
4. Serve in bowls and top with the remaining almonds. Decorate with a leaf of parsley, if you want.

Couscous Delight

Prep time: 5 min | **Cooking time**: 20 min | **Servings**: 4

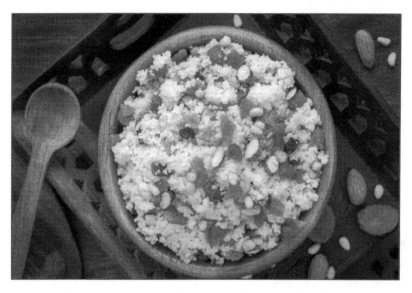

Nutritional Info (per serving):

- Calories – 310
- Fat – 9.7 g
- Fiber – 4.3 g
- Carbs – 51.2 g
- Protein – 9.5 g
- Sodium – 153 mg

Who said couscous is reserved for lunch or dinner? Enjoy this yummy breakfast that is very rich in fiber.

Ingredients:

- 1 cups soy milk
- 1 cinnamon stick
- 1 cup couscous, whole wheat uncooked
- 6 tsp brown sugar, divided
- ¼ cup currants, dried
- ½ cup apricots, dried and chopped
- 1 pinch salt
- ¼ cup almonds, crushed
- 1 tbsp pine nuts
- 4 tsp butter, melted and divided

Directions:

1. Put a saucepan over medium heat and pour in soy milk and the cinnamon stick. Let it heat for 3 minutes or until tiny bubbles start forming on the inner part of the pan, do not let it boil.
2. Remove the saucepan from the heat and stir in the couscous, 4 teaspoons of sugar, currants, apricots, and salt.
3. Put a lid on the saucepan and let it stand for 20 minutes. Remove the cinnamon stick.
4. Serve the couscous in 4 bowls and top each bowl with ½ teaspoon of sugar, 1 teaspoon of melted butter, crushed almonds, and pine nuts.
5. Serve hot.

Chapter 6: Mediterranean Pasta (Macaroni) Recipes

Penne Pasta with Pumpkin and Chili

Prep time: 10 min | **Cooking time**: 10 min | **Servings**: 4

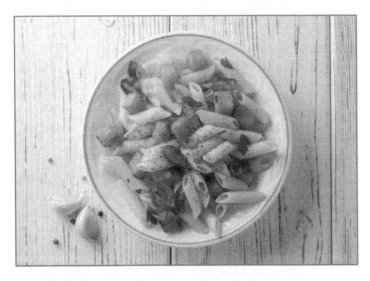

Nutritional Info (per serving):

- *Calories – 254*
- *Fat – 8.6 g*
- *Fiber – 3.7 g*
- *Carbs – 38.9 g*
- *Protein – 7.3 g*
- *Sodium – 304 mg*

A simple yet delicious dish for you to try.

Ingredients:

- 2 cups penne, cooked and drained
- 2 cups pumpkin, cubed
- 2 tbsp olive oil
- 1 clove garlic
- 1 tsp cayenne pepper, sliced
- ½ tsp salt
- ¼ tsp fresh ground black pepper
- 1 sprigs parsley, chopped

Directions:

1. In a saucepan, boil the pumpkin for 5-7 minutes until tender. Set aside.
2. In a medium heat pan, sauté the garlic in olive oil. Add the pumpkin and the cayenne. Sauté for 3 minutes.
3. In a bowl, place the penne and add the vegetable mixture on top. Toss until well blended.
4. Season with salt and pepper. Sprinkle with parsley.
5. Serve and enjoy.

Mediterranean Macaroni and Cheese

Prep time: 13 min | **Cooking time**: 30 min | **Servings**: 8

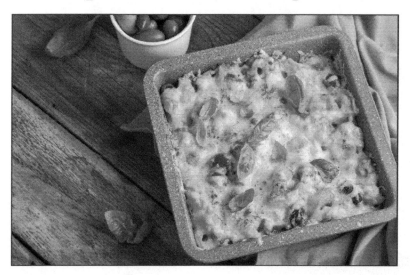

Nutritional Info (per serving):

- ✓ *Calories – 408*
- ✓ *Fat – 15.9 g*
- ✓ *Fiber – 3.1 g*
- ✓ *Carbs – 50.2 g*
- ✓ *Protein – 14.9 g*
- ✓ *Sodium – 450mg*

Ingredients:

- 14.5 oz tomatoes, diced
- ⅓ cup black or colorful olives, chopped
- 1 tbsp fresh basil, chopped
- ½ tsp oregano, dried
- 8 oz elbow macaroni pasta
- 2 tbsp butter
- 2 tbsp extra virgin olive oil
- ⅓ cup red onion, chopped
- 1 large clove garlic, minced
- 3 tbsp flour
- 2 cups whole milk
- 6 oz feta cheese, crumbled
- 2 oz mozzarella cheese, shredded
- ¼ tsp salt
- ¼ tsp ground black pepper

Directions:

1. In a bowl, mix the tomatoes, olives, basil, and oregano. Set aside.
2. Cook the macaroni according to the package. Drain well and set aside.
3. In medium heat pan, melt the butter in olive oil. Sauté the onion and garlic.
4. Add the tomato mixture and feta cheese. Let it simmer for 3 minutes.
5. Add the flour. Whisk the flour while slowly adding the milk to form the consistency of the sauce. Cook until thickened.
6. Grease the baking dish and place the macaroni and pour the sauce along with the macaroni.
7. Season with ground black pepper and salt. Top with mozzarella cheese.
8. Preheat your oven and bake it at 450°F for 20 to 25 minutes until top is golden brown.
9. Decorate with basil leaves. Serve and enjoy.

Chicken and Macaroni Baked

Prep time: 13 min | **Cooking time**: 1 hour | **Servings**: 8

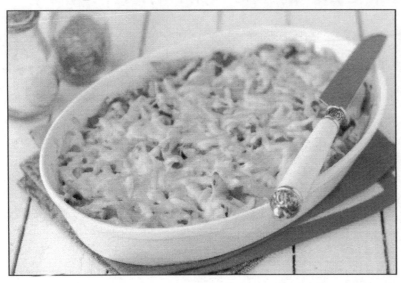

Nutritional Info (per serving):

- Calories – 441
- Fat – 18.7 g
- Fiber – 2.3 g
- Carbs – 47.3 g
- Protein – 21.3 g
- Sodium – 453mg

Ingredients:

- 2 cups penne macaroni, uncooked
- 2 cups chicken breast fillet, cut into strips
- 2 tbsp olive oil
- 1 large onion, finely chopped
- ½ cup carrot, finely chopped
- 2 cups zucchini, finely chopped, skin on
- 3 bacon rashers, chopped
- ½ cup tomato sauce
- ½ cup sour cream
- 1 ½ cup cheese, grated
- ½ tsp salt
- ¼ tsp ground black pepper

Directions:

1. In a saucepan, cook the macaroni in the boiling water until cooked. Drain and set aside.
2. In a large iron pan, heat olive oil and sear the chicken fillets for 7 to 10 minutes until cooked. Transfer cooked chicken fillets to a bowl.
3. In the same pan, stir-fry the vegetables: onion, carrot, and zucchini. Add the bacon and cook for 7 to 8 minutes.
4. Pour the tomato sauce and sour cream into the frying pan and let it simmer for 3 minutes.
5. In a baking dish, place the macaroni and the chicken, add the contents of the frying pan, and mix a little.
6. Season with salt and ground black pepper. Top with grated cheese.
7. Bake it at 360°F for 40 minutes or until the cheese is melted or brown.
8. Serve and enjoy.

Vermicelli Pudding

Prep time 7 min | **Cooking time**: 45 min | **Servings**: 2

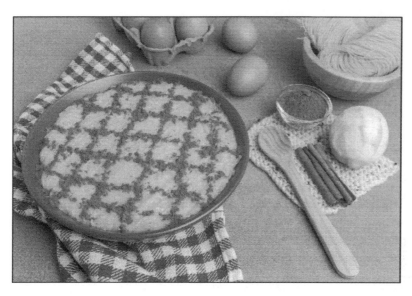

Nutritional Info (per serving):

- ✓ *Calories – 251*
- ✓ *Fat – 7.1 g*
- ✓ *Fiber – 0.9 g*
- ✓ *Carbs – 35.7 g*
- ✓ *Protein – 11.6 g*
- ✓ *Sodium – 120 mg*

Who said that pudding could not be done in a special way? Try this vermicelli pudding, and you will know the difference.

Ingredients:

- ½ cup vermicelli noodles
- 2 eggs
- 2 tbsp sugar
- 1 cup milk
- ½ cup sultanas
- ½ tsp vanilla essence
- ½ tsp nutmeg

Directions:

1. Cook the vermicelli according to the package instruction and drain it well.
2. In a bowl, whisk eggs with sugar and milk. Add vermicelli, sultanas, and vanilla and stir well.
3. Grease the baking dish and place the vermicelli mixture in it.
4. Bake vermicelli pudding at 320°F for 45 minutes.
5. Sprinkle with nutmeg on top. Serve and enjoy.

Baked Macaroni with Broccoli

Prep time: 13 min | **Cooking time**: 45 min | **Servings**: 4

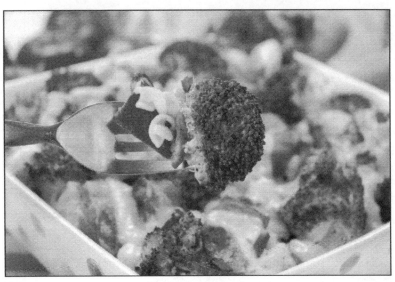

Nutritional Info (per serving):

- ✓ *Calories* – 381
- ✓ *Fat* – 22.8 g
- ✓ *Fiber* – 2.9 g
- ✓ *Carbs* – 34.8 g
- ✓ *Protein* – 11.9 g
- ✓ *Sodium* – 567 mg

A very delicious dish and easy to prepare for everybody.

Ingredients:

- 2 cups spiral macaroni, cooked and drained
- 2 tbsp olive oil
- 1 clove garlic, chopped
- 1 onion, chopped
- 1 cup red bell pepper, cut into strips
- 2 cups broccoli, sliced
- 1 cup mushrooms, thinly sliced
- ¾ cup sour cream
- ¾ cup water
- ¼ tsp salt
- ¼ tsp fresh ground black pepper
- ½ cup cheese, grated
- 1 sprigs parsley, chopped

Directions:

1. In a medium heat pan, sauté the garlic and onion in olive oil. Add the red bell pepper, broccoli, and the mushrooms. Cook for 3 minutes, stirring all along.
2. Add the water and sour cream and bring to a boil. Let it simmer for 4 minutes. Set aside.
3. In a baking dish, toss the macaroni with the broccoli mixture until well blended.
4. Season with salt and ground black pepper. Top with grated cheese.
5. Bake at 320°F for 45 minutes. Stir once halfway through cooking time.
6. Sprinkle with parsley for garnish.
7. Serve and enjoy.

Mediterranean Carbonara

Prep time: 7 min | **Cooking time**: 15 min | **Servings**: 8

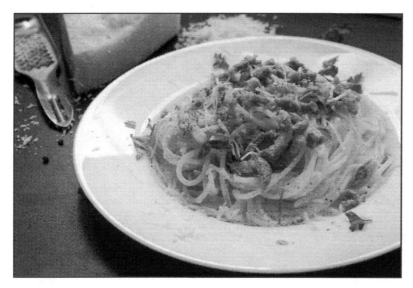

Nutritional Info (per serving):

- ✓ *Calories – 404*
- ✓ *Fat – 13.8 g*
- ✓ *Fiber – 0.9 g*
- ✓ *Carbs – 47.4 g*
- ✓ *Protein – 15.5 g*
- ✓ *Sodium – 355 mg*

An Italian classic, easy to prepare. Ideal for unexpected guest for a sure pleaser indeed.

Ingredients:

- 1 lbs whole-wheat spaghetti, dry
- 1 tbsp olive oil
- 1 onion, chopped
- 3 bacon rashers
- 2 eggs
- 2 egg yolk
- ½ cup sour cream
- 2 oz Parmesan, grated
- ½ tsp salt
- ¼ tsp ground black pepper
- 1 sprigs parsley, chopped

Directions:

1. Cook the spaghetti according to the package and drain it well. Set aside.
2. In medium heat pan, sauté onion in olive oil. Add bacon and fry until crisp.
3. Meanwhile, combine the egg, egg yolk, cream, and Parmesan in a bowl. Mix until well blended.
4. In medium heat pan, combine spaghetti with bacon and onion. Stir and cook for 2 minutes. Slowly pour the cream mixture. Season with salt and pepper to taste. Stir well and cook until ready.
5. Garnish with parsley. Serve and enjoy.

Pasta Salad

Prep time: 10 min | **Cooking time**: 8-10 min | **Servings**: 8

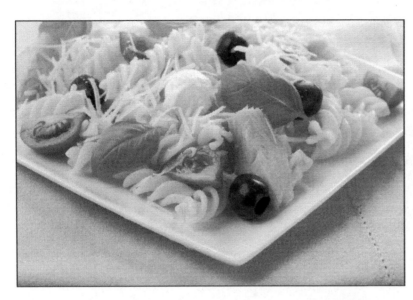

Nutritional Info (per serving):

- ✓ Calories – 241
- ✓ Fat – 9.8 g
- ✓ Fiber – 2.9 g
- ✓ Carbs – 26.2 g
- ✓ Protein – 12.9 g
- ✓ Sodium – 273 mg

A hearty salad ideal for every occasion and family reunions.

Ingredients:

- 8 oz macaroni
- 2 tbsp olive oil
- 2 tbsp fresh lemon juice
- 8 oz Mozzarella cheese, grated
- 8 oz artichoke hearts
- ½ cup olives
- ½ cup tomatoes quarter
- ¼ cup basil leaves

Directions:

1. Cook pasta for 8 minutes or according to the packet instructions without oil and salt.
2. Meanwhile, combine the olive oil and lemon juice and whisk well in a large bowl. Add the cheese, artichoke hearts and olives and toss well.
3. Drain the pasta once they are cooked. Do not run the pasta under cold water. Now add pasta to the mixture in the bowl and toss well.
4. Garnish with tomatoes and basil leaves. Serve at the room temperature.

Chapter 7: Mediterranean Meat and Poultry Recipes

Grilled Turkey Fillets

Prep time: 15 min | **Cooking time**: 30 minutes | **Servings**: 4

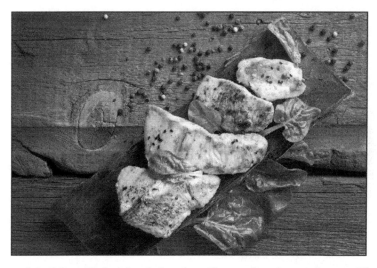

Nutritional Info (per serving):
- ✓ Calories – 168
- ✓ Fat – 7.9 g
- ✓ Fiber – 0.1 g
- ✓ Carbs – 1.0 g
- ✓ Protein – 22.1 g
- ✓ Sodium – 389 mg

A healthy dish ideal for family gatherings that will give your quality time extra special.

Ingredients:

- 1 lbs turkey fillets
- 1 tsp dried Italian seasoning
- ¼ tsp fresh ground black pepper
- ¼ tsp salt
- 1 tsp brown sugar
- 2 tbsp olive oil
- 1 tbsp lemon juice
- Basil leaves for garnish

Directions:

1. In a small bowl, combine Italian seasoning, fresh ground black pepper, salt, sugar, olive oil, and lemon juice until well blended.
2. Rub the turkey fillets with the resulting mixture and leave to marinate for 15 minutes.
3. Prepare the griller for medium-high heat. Grill the turkey fillets for 30 minutes until golden brown.
4. Serve with basil and enjoy.

Stuffed Peppers with Meat, Rice, and Vegetables

Prep time: 13 min | **Cooking time**: 30 min | **Servings**: 4

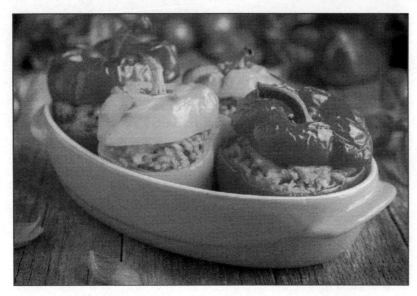

Nutritional Info (per serving):

- ✓ Calories – 459
- ✓ Fat – 8.5 g
- ✓ Fiber – 3.8 g
- ✓ Carbs – 87.5 g
- ✓ Protein – 8.3 g
- ✓ Sodium – 256mg

Ingredients:

- 2 tbsp olive oil
- 1 cloves garlic, minced
- 1 onion, diced
- 1 medium carrot, finely diced
- 1 lbs ground pork
- 2 cups cooked rice
- ½ tbsp dried Italian seasoning
- ¼ tsp kosher salt
- 4 large bell peppers
- ½ cup water

Directions:

1. In medium heat pan, sauté the garlic and onion in olive oil.
2. Add the carrot and sauté another 3 minutes.
3. Add the ground pork and cook for 6-7 minutes, stirring the meat and breaking up the lumps.
4. Add the pre-cooked rice and salt. Season with Italian seasoning and mix well. Then remove the pan from the heat, let it cool a little.
5. Cut the top of each bell pepper and scoop out the seeds. Retain tops for later use.
6. Stuff the bell peppers with rice and meat mixture and cover with pepper tops.
7. In a baking dish, arrange the stuffed bell peppers. Carefully pour water between the peppers into the baking dish. Bake it at 450°F preheated oven for 30 minutes.
8. Serve and enjoy.

Delicious Chicken Breasts with Lemon

Prep time: 7 min | **Cooking time**: 25 min | **Servings**: 3

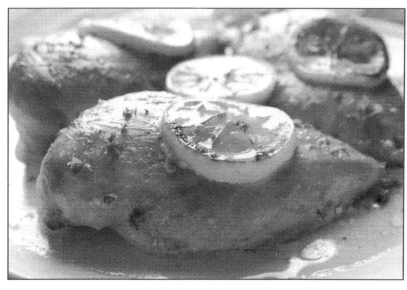

Nutritional Info (per serving):

- *Calories – 361*
- *Fat – 24.2 g*
- *Fiber – 2.6 g*
- *Carbs – 22.1 g*
- *Protein – 15.2 g*
- *Sodium – 463mg*

Simple yet delicious chicken meal that is a sure star on every dinner table.

Ingredients:

- 3 chicken breast fillet
- 2 tbsp olive oil
- 2 tsp unsalted butter
- 1 clove garlic, minced
- 1 onion, diced
- 1 lemon, sliced
- ¼ tsp salt
- ¼ tsp fresh ground black pepper
- ½ tsp thyme, dried
- ¼ cup chicken broth
- 2 tbsp lemon juice
- 1 tsp fresh parsley, chopped

Directions:

1. In a medium heat pan, melt the butter in olive oil and sauté the garlic and the onion.
2. Season the chicken breasts with fresh ground black pepper and salt and sear it both sides until golden brown. Add the lemon slices.
3. Transfer the chicken breasts to the serving dish.
4. In the same frying pan pour the broth, lemon juice and add dried thyme. Let it simmer for 3-4 minutes until thickened.
5. Pour the sauce over chicken breasts. Garnish with lemon slices and fresh parsley.
6. Serve and enjoy.

Roasted Lamb with Vegetables

Prep time: 7 min | **Cooking time**: 1 hour | **Servings**: 4

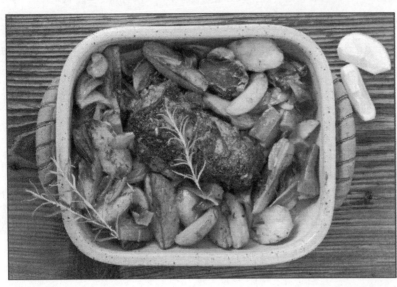

Nutritional Info (per serving):

- ✓ *Calories – 362*
- ✓ *Fat – 15.9 g*
- ✓ *Fiber – 3.8 g*
- ✓ *Carbs – 20.9 g*
- ✓ *Protein – 33.6 g*
- ✓ *Sodium – 260mg*

Ingredients:

- 1 lbs lamb, leg shanks
- ½ tbsp dried Italian seasoning
- ¼ tsp salt
- ¼ tsp fresh ground black pepper
- 2 tbsp olive oil
- 1 cloves garlic, minced
- 1 onion, quartered
- 2 medium carrots, cut into ¼ inch strips
- 1 medium potato, quartered
- 2 apple, quartered
- 2 sprigs fresh rosemary to garnish

Directions:

1. Season the lamb shanks with Italian seasoning, salt, and fresh ground black pepper.
2. Preheat oven to 370°F. Place lamb into the greased baking dish, cover with a foil and bake it for 40 minutes.
3. Meanwhile, in medium heat pan, sauté the garlic and onion in olive oil.
4. Add the carrots and potatoes, and sauté for another 3-5 minutes.
5. Transfer vegetables to the baking dish around the lamb and add the apples.
6. Bake the lamb with vegetables for another 20 minutes without foil until golden brown outside and tender inside.
7. Garnish with fresh rosemary. Serve and enjoy.

Pan Fried Pork Chops with Orange Sauce

Prep time: 5 min | **Cooking time**: 20 min | **Servings**: 8

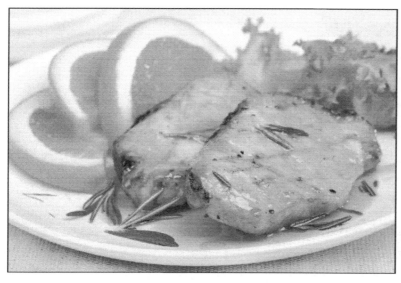

Nutritional Info (per serving):

- Calories – 412
- Fat – 31.7 g
- Fiber – 0.6 g
- Carbs – 4.5 g
- Protein – 25.8 g
- Sodium – 297mg

This dish will give your guest a burst of the orange and delicious taste of pork chop.

Ingredients:

- 2 lbs pork chops, lean, boneless
- ¾ tsp salt
- ½ tsp fresh ground black pepper
- 2 tbsp olive oil
- 1 cloves garlic, minced
- ½ cup of freshly squeezed orange juice
- 1 orange, wedged

Directions:

1. Sprinkle the pork chops with salt and fresh ground black pepper.
2. In a medium heat pan, sauté the garlic in olive oil.
3. Add the pork chops and sear it on both sides until tender and golden brown. Remove fried pork chops from the pan and set aside.
4. In the same pan, pour the orange juice. Let it simmer for 4 minutes until the sauce thickens.
5. In a serving plate, place the pork chops with orange sauce and orange wedges.
6. Serve and enjoy.

Mediterranean Meatballs in Tomato Sauce

Prep time: 6 min | **Cooking time**: 35 min | **Servings**: 4

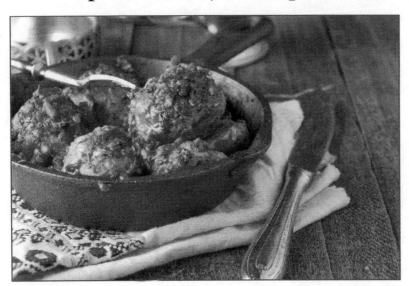

Nutritional Info (per serving):

- ✓ Calories – 320
- ✓ Fat – 9.0 g
- ✓ Fiber – 4.3 g
- ✓ Carbs – 20.8 g
- ✓ Protein – 38.7 g
- ✓ Sodium – 480mg

Ingredients:

- 1 lbs ground beef
- 1 tsp dried Italian seasoning
- 1 cloves garlic, minced
- 1 onion, finely chopped
- ½ cup whole-grain flour
- 1 medium carrot, grated
- 2 tbsp olive oil
- 4 medium tomatoes, chopped
- ⅓ cup broth
- 1 tsp cornstarch
- ½ tsp salt
- ¼ tsp ground black pepper
- 1 tsp fresh parsley, chopped

Directions:

1. In a bowl, combine the ground beef, Italian seasoning, garlic, onion, flour, and carrot until well blended.
2. Scoop one tablespoon of meat mixtures and carefully form a ball. Set aside.
3. In a high heat pan, deep fry the meatballs in olive oil until golden brown.
4. Repeat until all the meatballs are cooked. Set aside.
5. In a boiling pan, simmer the broth with tomatoes for 15 minutes.
6. Add the cornstarch to thicken the sauce. Season with salt and pepper.
7. Transfer the meatballs to the sauce, top with sauce and parsley and let rest for 5 to 10 minutes.
8. Serve and enjoy.

Chapter 8: Mediterranean Desserts Recipes

Honey Glazed Apple

Prep time: 3 min | **Cooking time**: 7-8 min | **Servings**: 4

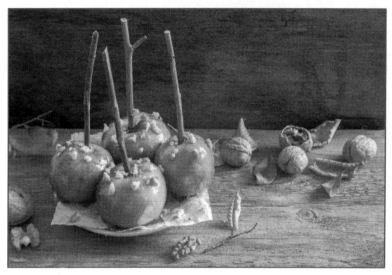

Nutritional Info (per serving):

- ✓ Calories – 264
- ✓ Fat – 2.8 g
- ✓ Fiber – 5.7 g
- ✓ Carbs – 63.7 g
- ✓ Protein – 1.8 g
- ✓ Sodium – 3 mg

A perfect dessert for every occasion. A honey glazed apple will give your guest a sweet reward.

Ingredients:

- 4 apples
- ½ cup sugar
- ¼ cup water
- ½ cup orange juice
- 1 tbsp honey
- 2 tbsp walnut, crushed

Directions:

1. In a low-heat pan, slowly caramelize the sugar in the water.
2. Add the orange juice and honey to the caramel. Bring to boil. Let it simmer on low for 1 to 2 minutes until thickened, stirring all the time.
3. Dip the apple into the warm caramel mixture. Stab the stick into the apple through its heart. Sprinkle on top with the crushed walnut.
4. Serve and enjoy.

Honey-Nuts Baked Pears

Prep time: 7 min | **Cooking time**: 25 min | **Servings**: 6

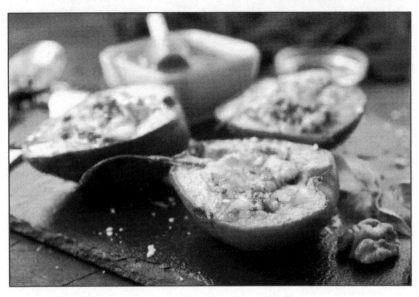

Nutritional Info (per serving):

- ✓ *Calories – 146*
- ✓ *Fat – 6.2 g*
- ✓ *Fiber – 3.2 g*
- ✓ *Carbs – 22.1 g*
- ✓ *Protein – 3.2 g*
- ✓ *Sodium – 15 mg*

A dessert for everyone that loves pears in a special way.

Ingredients:

- 3 ripe medium pears, peeled, halved, and cored
- ¼ cup pear nectar
- 2 tbsp honey
- 1 tsp butter
- 1 tbsp orange zest
- ½ cup mascarpone cheese
- ⅓ cup crushed walnuts
- 2 tsp powdered sugar

Directions:

1. In a small bowl, mix pear nectar, honey, and butter.
2. In a baking dish, arrange the pears and pour the honey mixture over each pear.
3. Bake the pears in 350°F preheated oven for 10 minutes.
4. In a bowl, combine the orange zest, mascarpone cheese, walnuts, and powdered sugar.
5. Stuff pears with cheese mixture and bake for another 15 minutes.
6. Serve and enjoy.

Strawberry Chocolate Dip

Prep time: 7 min | **Cooking time**: 15 min | **Servings**: 8

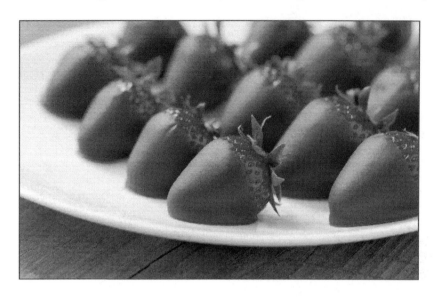

Nutritional Info (per serving):

- ✓ Calories – 164
- ✓ Fat – 8.3 g
- ✓ Fiber – 3.0 g
- ✓ Carbs – 21.2 g
- ✓ Protein – 2.4 g
- ✓ Sodium – 18mg

An ideal dish for everyone especially who have a steady day ahead.

Ingredients:

- 2 lbs strawberries, with calyxes and stalks
- 1 cup dark chocolate
- 1 tbsp olive oil

Directions:

1. In a double boiling pan, place the chocolates in the heatproof bowl. Slowly melt the chocolates.
2. Stir the olive oil into the melted chocolates and let it cool down.
3. Gently take each strawberry by the stalk and dip it on all sides into the melted chocolate. Transfer to the parchment paper. Cool in the refrigerator before serving.
4. Serve and enjoy.

Vegan Blueberry Vanilla Smoothie

Prep time: 3 min | **Cooking time**: 1 min | **Servings**: 2

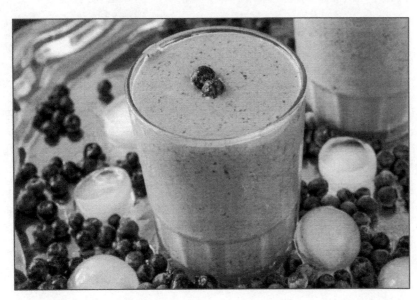

Nutritional Info (per serving):

- ✓ Calories – 233
- ✓ Fat – 19.2 g
- ✓ Fiber – 3.2 g
- ✓ Carbs – 15.7 g
- ✓ Protein – 2.2 g
- ✓ Sodium – 13 mg

An ideal dish for everyone especially who have a steady day ahead.

Ingredients:

- ²/₃ cup of almond milk
- ²/₃ cup of blueberries, frozen
- 1 tsp of pure vanilla extract
- 1 tbsp of agave nectar

Directions:

1. Put almond milk, blueberries, vanilla extract, and agave nectar in a blender and process until smooth.
2. You can add more agave depending on how sweet you want your smoothie to be.
3. Serve immediately.

Chapter 9:
7-Day Mediterranean Diet Meal Plan to Lose Weight

This 7-day plan is ideal for people who want to lose weight in a manner that they can still enjoy the food that they love but in moderation.

This meal plan is calculated for the daily caloric intake limited to 1200 kcal per a day. It is suitable for a person who is physically low-active. In total, you have five meals a day: three main and two additional. Generally, the main meals contain 300 calories each, and two snacks for 150 calories.

Drink more than 2 liters of water, exclude sweet and sodas drinks. Eat a lot of fruit and fresh vegetables.

If you are physically active and go in for sports, then you need a nutrition plan of 1500-1600 kcal. The daily caloric intake must differ depending on the relation to your physical activity and individual health. It is much better to use personalized menus for your individual needs to lose weight with pleasure and with health benefits. Please always consult a licensed professional before making changes to your lifestyle or diet.

Day 1

	kcal	Page
Breakfast	**215**	
Oatmeal with Strawberry	135	42
1 medium apple	80	
Snack	**118**	
Caprese Salad	118	18
Lunch	**391**	
Delicious Chicken Breasts with Lemon	361	56
2 ripe tomatoes	30	
Snack	**45**	
½ cup fresh cherries	45	
Dinner	**436**	
Seafood Paella	351	44
1 glass (100 g) of red wine	85	
Total calories	**1205**	

Day 2

	kcal	Page
Breakfast	**296**	
Garbanzos Greek Hummus	206	41
1 slice whole grain bread	90	
Snack	**86**	
1 orange	86	
Lunch	**419**	
Roasted Garlic Butter Salmon	294	40
Colorful Vegetable Salad	125	24
Snack	**50**	
½ pomegranate	50	
Dinner	**350**	
Mediterranean Meatballs in Tomato Sauce	320	59
3 tbsp pitted Kalamata olives OR 2 ripe tomatoes	30	
Total calories	**1201**	

Day 3

	kcal	Page
Breakfast	**344**	
Quinoa Heaven	344	45
Snack	**80**	
1 pear	80	
Lunch	**358**	
Salmon Steak Fillet with Cheese Crust Breading	323	33
1 ripe tomato	15	
1 medium baby cucumber	15	
5 leaves of lettuce	5	
Snack	**105**	
2 medium plums	60	
1 medium fresh fig	45	
Dinner	**312**	
Fresh Green Salad with Shrimps and Avocado	133	20
1 slice whole-grain nut bread	120	
Greek Yogurt Dip	59	17
Total calories	**1199**	

Day 4

	kcal	Page
Breakfast	**251**	
Vermicelli Pudding	251	50
Snack	**60**	
1 peach	60	
Lunch	**471**	
Baked Salmon with Lemon and Cherry Tomatoes	346	39
Colorful Vegetable Salad	125	24
Snack	**35**	
1 clementine	35	
Dinner	**385**	
Stuffed Eggplant with Fried Vegetables	385	26
Total calories	**1202**	

Day 5

	kcal	Page
Breakfast	**310**	
Couscous Delight	310	46
Snack	**62**	
1 cup grapes	62	
Lunch	**459**	
Stuffed Peppers with Meat, Rice, and Vegetables	459	55
Snack	**33**	
1 ripe tomato	15	
1 medium baby cucumber	15	
3 leaves of lettuce	3	
Dinner	**339**	
Baked Salmon with Vegetables Ratatouille	339	32
Total calories	**1203**	

Day 6

	kcal	Page
Breakfast	**324**	
Baked Beans	183	43
1 boiled egg	72	
1 slice whole wheat bread	69	
Snack	**154**	
Shrimps and Vegetables Stir-Fry	154	37
Lunch	**347**	
Grilled Turkey Fillets	168	54
Moroccan Style Vegetable Stew	179	28
Snack	**49**	
1 cup sliced strawberries	49	
Dinner	**326**	
Pasta Salad	241	53
1 glass (100 g) of red wine	85	
Total calories	**1200**	

Day 7

	kcal	Page
Breakfast	**326**	
Bulgur salad	326	23
Snack	**91**	
Eggplant Rolls Stuffed with Cream Cheese and Tomatoes	91	15
Lunch	**381**	
Baked Macaroni with Broccoli	381	51
Snack	**70**	
1 cup pineapple chunks	70	
Dinner	**331**	
Grilled Sea Bass with Parsley and Lemon	296	36
1 ripe tomato	15	
1 medium baby cucumber	15	
5 leaves of lettuce	5	
Total calories	**1199**	

CONCLUSION

Thanks for downloading this book and reading all the way to the end. We hope that this recipe book would be a great help to your endeavor toward tasteful and healthy living.

Made in the USA
San Bernardino, CA
05 January 2019